Strength in a Heartbeat

Diary of a Heart Transplant Story

A Second Chance at Life

by Lynne Robitaille

Dedication

This book is dedicated to the angel who decided to become an organ donor. You saved my daughter's life.

With many thanks,

To my son Michael, his wife Katie and my granddaughter Madison, for all of your unconditional love and support and for the many, many trips you all made to Boston, just to take me out to dinner. That will never be forgotten.

To my sister Donna, for all the help and guidance you gave us through the worst time of our lives.

To my husband Dean, for your love and the encouragement to write our story. Love you, Sweetheart

Edited by Sutton Mason

Published : August 2017

Made in the USA

Content

Helpful Suggestions if You Find Yourself Living in a Hospital

I have included in the back of the book, some helpful suggestions, if you find yourself spending a long period of time in a hospital setting. I had to find this out as our days went by.
I hope this will help, Remember not all institutions are the same, each others different amenities.

Introduction

This book is a true, real life account of what it is like to hear "your daughter's heart is failing; we are going to place her on the transplant list." The journey we were on is nothing like what you see in the movies. I wish it were. Nothing really prepared us for what our lives would be like for nearly a year and a half. The doctor's favorite motto was "this is not a sprint, it's a marathon." Boy, did we learn that.

My name is Lynne Robitaille and my daughter, Lauren Mezzo is a heart transplant recipient. Lauren was placed on the transplant list on March 13, 2013. She received her gift of life, a new heart, on December 30, 2013 at Brigham and Women's Hospital in Boston, Massachusetts.

When Lauren was born on May 24, 1990, the doctors told me I had a beautiful, healthy baby girl. I was the happiest person in the world. Eight years earlier on November 13, 1982 I gave birth to my beautiful son, Mikey. When I gave birth to Michael, it was a very hard labor. He ended up turning himself and was a breach baby. Eventually they had to perform a C-section to get him out safely.

Michael is a healthy young man now with a family of his own. My marriage ended with his father when he was 5 years old. I could say the reason was we were young, I was only 20 years old when we were married. Mikey has a great relationship with his father, hell, I can say we all do. Michael Sr. joins us in family occasions. I remarried in 1999 to a wonderful man Dean Robitaille Sr. In our family we do not use the word step, mother or father. Lauren was five years old at the time, she calls him her Fosha. As for her biological father, we have agreed to say not, in the picture.

When I gave birth to Lauren she was a scheduled C-section. The reason for that was the trouble I'd had with her brother; I didn't want to take any chances with any problems. I already had my son and now a daughter; a mother's dream.

As Lauren was growing up, she was a healthy, strong little girl progressing normally for a child her age, until she turned ten.

Then our world changed.

I feel compelled to share our journey not only to provide a true testimony as to what life is like going through this process, but also in hopes that it may give support to others. There are thousands of people currently awaiting transplants; men, women and children waiting for donated organs such as hearts, pancreases, kidneys, livers, lungs and intestines. Tissue is needed to replace bone, tendons and ligaments lost to trauma, cancer and other diseases. Corneas are needed to restore sight, skin grafts to heal burn patients. The list goes on.

Living in a hospital is hard. It's very hard. Not only for the patient but also for a family member that chooses to stay there. I chose to stay. Not everyone does. I would like you to know, if you are living in a hospital now, please do not feel alone.

I started this book based on the journal I kept throughout our journey. The diary helped to keep loved ones informed whereas I found it very hard to call my family all the time; it was emotionally draining to talk,

so writing made it easier to express, inform and even bitch, when I needed to.

I have also included a few tips on how to survive living in a hospital; there are many programs available that no one tells you about. This is a true story; the story of my daughter's heart transplant and the time we were forced to live in a hospital.

Chapter 1

How it All Started

As I'm sitting here trying to figure out when this nightmare began, my mind is just so flooded with different thoughts. For the past 14 years, our lives have been nothing but normal. This is not a life I expected nor would I ever want my child to have to go through. I'll be honest; I was in such denial. I would hear what the doctors would tell us but didn't want to believe it.

My daughter Lauren wrote a paper in college at Mount Ida College in Newton, Massachusetts. She was studying to become a veterinary assistant. To try to explain how it all started, Lauren wrote the following……

Strength

Strength. Strength holds different definitions depending upon the person. One may reply that the definition of "strength" has to do with how physically strong an individual is, whereas someone else may reply with a mental aspect or the ability to cope with difficult situations. Growing up, I always heard, "Lauren, you're one of the strongest people I know." Honestly, I'm not a body builder nor are my biceps and triceps extremely muscular, but I do indeed have strength.

Ever since I was a little girl, I knew I was not like all my friends. I was special or "rare." From kindergarten to eighth grade, I attended the same Catholic school. My school was no more than four hundred or so, making it easy to know everyone else's business all the time. Keeping up with the other kids in gym class was always a challenge. I was not a lazy child; I rode horses and loved playing outside but when it came to physical strength tests, I would get embarrassed. Nationally, once a child hits fourth grade they are tested in various components of physical activity and endurance. I will always remember this one instance in gym when it came time to do sit-ups. I held my partner's feet as she exceeded the amount needed to qualify for the Presidential Award. It was now my turn. I laid down, bent my knees, and placed my hands behind my head. I'd never really attempted a sit-up, so I had no idea about what was about to happen. The teacher blew the whistle and everyone began. "One, two, three…" I could hear the other children shouting in the gymnasium but my partner was silent. I could not do it. I could not pick my head up off the blue mat. Tears began to fill my eyes as the teacher said "and stop!" I ran into the locker room crying my eyes out as my friends chased me saying "maybe it's because your brain is so heavy cause you're so smart?"

About six months later, I went for my yearly check-up at the doctor. She ran through her usual procedures. I always knew I had asthma so I was not surprised when she checked my lungs and heard wheezing. From there, she took her stetho-

scope to my heart and heard a slight murmur. Checking my eyes, ears, throat and so on, she continued. The doctor then had me do something I had never done before. She asked me to bend forward, as if to touch my toes. She ran her fingers down my vertebrae and could noticeably tell that my right shoulder blade was higher than my left. The look upon her face made my parents and I worry. It was at that moment that my life changed forever.

Within three months I was diagnosed with scoliosis and a heart murmur. I was an eleven-year-old girl dealing with puberty and just trying to find myself when I was hit with the news that for the next few years of my life I would need to wear a back brace. I'd never heard of such a thing; a curvature of the spine. The top of my spine measured 30" to the right while the lower curvature measured 14" to the left. Twenty hours a day, seven days a week, for four and a half years, I was trapped inside my brace, the plastic shell that held me together. My parents and I were informed that the brace would not cure or straighten my spine but rather prevent it from worsening since they were not sure which form of scoliosis I had. I felt alone.

My health just began to turn into a domino effect. My doctor said she was concerned about my heart murmur and I was sent to a cardiologist for further testing. My cardiologist ran test after test to determine the severity of the leakage in my heart. EKG's, ultra sounds, and stress tests became a necessity for my cardiovascular appointments. I felt like a guinea pig, a test subject being used for science. By the age of eleven, I was already taking eight pills a day. The madness did not stop there.

Since I was having problems in my heart, the most important muscle in the body, my doctor felt it important that the rest of my muscles be checked. Shriners Hospital in Springfield, MA soon became my second home. It took multiple visits, tests, and x-rays to only hear more bad news. During the spring of fifth grade, I was diagnosed with Muscular Dystrophy. This helped answer the question as to why I could not walk on my heels, touch my chin to my chest, or why I had such great difficulty a year prior in doing a sit-up. The emotional distress I was going through was unimaginable.

As time passed, I no longer fit in the criteria for Muscular Dystrophy. A biopsy was performed on my right thigh, leaving a one-inch inch scar to add to my memories. The testing came back with no answers. It looked normal but I clearly was not the typical child in front of my doctors. Questions were going unanswered, hope was fading, and tears were forming. No longer could I only rely on the technology of Western Massachusetts. A hospital in Boston turned into my new friend. The doctors in Boston suggested new approaches for tackling my health problems. I tried wearing leg braces for a few months but found no benefit from doing so. I had little hope.

Even though my school was little, I still faced the ridicule. People would always draw attention to my posture began to form. I was known as "the girl with the back brace," some insisting I was a cripple, while others just found enjoyment in staring. From wearing my back brace for such a long period of time during my growing years, the muscles in my back began to tighten up and worsen. I had no need to use them since my body was held together by a girdle of plastic. To this day, my back brace has left a miserable mark upon me in the form of poor posture. It is important for me to comfortably stand up straight and tall. When I try, the combination of the muscle disease in my neck and the result of wearing the back brace make it difficult to hold my head, breathe or swallow.

The past eight years of my life have been spent in and out of doctors' offices. My pill count has gone up to fourteen a day. I have participated in numerous studies and have worn three different bracing devices from my back to the trial and error of my leg braces. Currently, I wear a brace around my neck from time to time to stretch my neck muscles. My journey is far from over. To this day, I still have great difficulty with every day activities. Walking produces a great amount of pain in my neck. This results in me having to hold my neck in a forward position, otherwise it will fall back. A great amount of pain also presents itself in my lower back as well.

It was not until this past February that one of my usual doctors suggested I see a geneticist. No other doctor had recommended this idea in the past, so I thought it was worth a try. This sent my family and I on another journey to Boston. Blood samples were taken from my parents and me and sent to a laboratory to be tested. Two months later, the results were in and another appointment scheduled. I could finally tell people who questioned what was wrong with me, what I really had.

In April, I was finally properly diagnosed with a very rare muscle disease called Laing Distal Myopathy (LDM). Isolation and loneliness set in. It is a one in a million disease that affects the dorsiflexors of the toes, ankles, and fingers. LDM also affects the neck and heart. When I found out, I had mixed feelings. I was happy that I finally had a legitimate name for the disease that had been causing me such hardship for over eight years, but then at the same time, I lost hope. My muscle disease is not like breast cancer in the sense of research and cures. Few people possess what I have, therefore the research is slow and not a priority. I can now live my life though, knowing that I will not die young due to this genetic disease. From my un-

derstanding, my DNA does not line up properly toward the ends of the strand, causing the mutation. With this said, before considering ever giving birth to a child, my best option to avoid passing it to my offspring would be testing one of the cells to see whether or not Laing Distal Myopathy is present. From there, it would be my choice whether to abort the baby.

My health problems have caused me tremendous emotional problems. The summer before going into my freshman year of high school was when I first sought counseling. I spent a majority of the year suffering from depression. Bouncing around between four different therapists, thoughts of suicide passed through my head from time to time but I knew I did not have it in me to take my own life.

I have learned to play the hand I was dealt with skill. I believe it has made me the caring and understanding person I am today. I try not to take the simple things in life for granted because you never know when you may lose them. It is still impossible for me to stand up straight and my self-esteem is effected greatly by this but I think of everything I can do. No longer do I suffer from depression or suicidal thoughts. You only live once, why not make the best of it? I still do cry and get upset occasionally but I always think that there are people out there who have it far worse than I do.

Strength. I have always been told I am a strong person for everything I have gone through thus far in my short life. I carry the word with me everywhere I go. I wear a necklace that has a circular pendant with "Strength" engraved in it representing that I have what it takes to overcome anything thrown at me. Three

days after I turned eighteen I went to a tattoo parlor, handed over $140 and signed my name on the dotted line. I knew for a while I permanently wanted

"Strength" upon my body. My muscle weaknesses gave me the mental strength to overcome the obstacles thrown in my way along this path we call life.

Lauren Meizo
December 8, 2008

After reading Lauren's account, one may wonder what else one person could possibly deal with. Everyone obviously has obstacles they have to overcome in a lifetime but we never could have imagined a life threatening heart transplant in our lives. You always hear that expression "life isn't fair," and I tend to agree.

There is no greater pain than watching your child suffer through so many different medical problems. With denial in the back of my mind, I kept thinking *no, this is not happening, she'll get better.*

Then reality really set in and I had to gather all my strength for the long road we were heading down.

Chapter 2

When You Hear the Words "Heart Failure"

At the age of 22 years old in October of 2012, Lauren was complaining she was experiencing shortness of breath when she would lie down, feeling very fatigued and experiencing abdominal pains. Taking her to the local emergency room, they ran a few tests and admitted her to the hospital for what they'd concluded was a case of pneumonia. Since she now had a cardiologist in Boston, I expressed our concern that we wanted to inform her doctors in Boston of her condition. I only really trusted Lauren's cardiologist in Boston at this point. The reason for thinking like this, one of Lauren's cardiologist here actually told us to go to Boston. They are more advanced in technology and education with new treatments. So from that moment on, the only cardiologist we trusted was in Boston.

After a few days in the hospital, Lauren was feeling better. When she was released, we had a follow up appointment in Boston. While her lungs were clear, she still wasn't feeling well. She was feeling bloated which meant she was retaining fluids. She had regained a couple of pounds, we didn't think too much of it, but her cardiologist was concerned about her weight gain and the pressure she was experiencing in her chest.

We live in Chicopee, Massachusetts so this meant a road trip, 90 miles from here to Boston. Off we went. Fill the car with gas, money for tolls and tips to the valet at the hospital. My husband took the day off to go to this appointment with us. That made me feel better because I just might need to lean on him.

As they ran the routine tests, an EKG indicated that the pressure on the right side of her heart was elevated a bit. Adjusting her medications, the doctor told us to keep our eyes open for any type of weight gain or shortness of breath.

For the next two months, everything seemed to be going fine. A few days before Christmas, Lauren said she couldn't breathe and she felt heaviness in her chest. We went straight to the local emergency room and she was once again admitted. She was placed in the ICU, where we were told they'd discovered fluid build-up around her heart.

As a mother, I looked around the room wondering what in the world was going on. *Why is this happening?* I thought. We knew Lauren had something different going on with her heart but this was really turning into something very real. Up to this point, I'd been in denial that this would ever be a possible reality. Having a rare muscle disease was bad enough, but now her heart…

When Lauren was admitted to the hospital, not being in a private room, I looked around to assess how I could best sleep there with her. As with most hospital rooms, it seemed a chair would be my only option. Understandably, Lauren was very scared and nervous but I assured her she was not alone; I was staying. The hospital wanted me to leave, but that wasn't happening. My daughter needed me and there was no way I was leaving. Mom won.

Lauren was diressed in order for intravenous medication to be given to help rid her body of extra fluid around her heart. With Christmas only five days away, we kept wondering if we were going to be spending the holidays in a hospital room. This was the beginning to our worst nightmare. At this point, it had begun to sink in that my daughter was starting to get very sick. Her health aside, I couldn't even imagine the thought of spending Christmas in the hospital.

With her medications adjusted yet again, we were discharged on Christmas Eve around 5 p.m. I kept thinking someone had answered my prayers to be home for the holiday. That evening, it felt so good to finally sit on the couch after having spent so many hours in a hospital room, especially after having to sleep in a chair. My husband Dean and I just sat there exhausted; drained but relieved our family was home for Christmas. But we both knew it wasn't over. We knew this was just the beginning after having been hospitalized twice in such a short period of time. It was time to find the strength within us to be there for whatever was to come.

After the holidays, we spoke with Lauren's cardiologist in Boston and she suggested she be seen by a heart failure specialist.

On January 16, 2013 we drove to Brigham and Women's Hospital in Boston. I remember the car ride as being very quiet. I think the only words spoken were when my husband said, "Do you have the toll money ready?" We all had the same thoughts going through our minds but we didn't want to say them aloud.

Lauren wasn't feeling well, complaining of stomach pains and a heavy chest. Arriving at the hospital, I had a feeling that we weren't going home that day. *My daughter isn't feeling well and we're meeting a new doctor,* I told myself.

As we sat in the examining room waiting for the doctor, we didn't know what to expect. They did the standard EKG and told us the doctor would be in shortly. Looking around the sterile exam room, I felt as if I'd been kicked in the stomach; I had a pretty good idea as to what was coming. Hearing the knock on the door, I knew our lives were about to change forever.

The doctor examined Lauren's jugular venous pressure (on the right side of her neck) with trained eyes and EKG results in hand. Looking at us earnestly, she claimed, "Lauren is in congestive heart failure and I need to admit her today." Tears quickly filled my eyes, my body numbing. Looking to Dean, he was in the same state of disbelief. Turning to Lauren, I think she felt a little relieved to finally be able to have an answer as to why she way feeling the way she had been.

> Heart Failure. What?! Heart Failure. What, are you serious? My daughter is in heart failure. What is that?

To hear those words, the rest of the world just disappears. For so many years, every time we went to the doctors, all I remember is crying on our way home. *Dear Lord, why?* Then you pull yourself together and say "okay, we'll handle this and do what we need to do to get her better." It was now time to start doing homework on Congestive Heart Failure. (CHF)

**Congestive Heart Failure, or CHF, is a life treating disease that occurs when your heart becomes too weak to pump blood properly. It is caused by damage to the heart. Over time, the damage causes the heart to work harder and grow larger. The harder your heart works, the weaker it becomes until it cannot work properly.*
CHF cannot be cured, however there are many things you can do to keep it from getting worse. In heart failure, your heart cannot pump enough oxygen-rich blood to the rest of the body; this is especially true when you exercise or are active. This causes a shortage of oxygen and nutrients in the blood, which can make you feel weak and tired.
*When your heart is not pumping effectively it can also cause blood to back up in your body. The back-up causes fluid to leak from your vessels and into the tissues. This is called congestion: congestion can make it hard to breathe, causing swelling in the ankles and legs and it will make you feel full and not want to eat**

Chapter 3

Longest Doctor Appointment
January 16, 2013 - Cardiac Specialist, Boston Ma.

In my wildest dreams I would have never imagined that I would always remember this date. This was the day our whole world fell apart. As I looked around the examining room, looking at my daughter, I held my husband's hand, not even able to imagine what was going through Lauren's mind. We were told years ago that someday, just possibly, Lauren might need a heart transplant, but is that what she was thinking about? I could only guess because it was crossing my mind and I know Dean was thinking about it too.

I kept telling myself, *don't start thinking the worse, she's going to be okay. We're in one of the world's best hospitals, with the best doctors.* Lauren's doctor informed us that she'd ordered a room, then went on to explain how her body was retaining fluid. The plan is to use aggressive dieresis; the diuretics Lauren had been taking at home weren't working, so she needed to be on an IV drip.

After being given so much information, our next question was, "how long will we be here?" I was wondering if it was just overnight or a longer stay, since we didn't pack anything. We were told she wasn't sure but at least a week for the amount of fluid that Lauren was carrying. Our only responsibility at home was our 12-year-old Yellow

Lab, Ralf; the best puppy you could ask for. We only needed to make arrangements for him.

What do we do now? While Boston is only two hours from our home, it felt a million miles away. First thing my husband Dean did was call work, being a Wednesday he was taking the rest of the week off. He said there was no way he was leaving us. Lauren was scared; I told her that I would not leave the hospital, we would leave together. The hospital told us that being a cardiac patient Lauren will be in the Shapiro Building. This part of the hospital was new and all the rooms were private so Dean and I would be able to stay with her.

It seemed like forever before the hospital had a room available for Lauren. While we were waiting, I called my son Mike to inform him of his sister's condition. He asked us what we needed from home and all I could do was stand there, my mind blank. *What do we need?* After providing him with a list, he assured us he would be up the next day. One person I can always count on is my son Mikey. Whatever we need, he's always there for his family. He's one of the good ones. Family first.

Our appointment had been at 10:30am and by 3pm we were on our way to Lauren's room. Walking down the corridor, giving shy smiles to passersby in the hallway, all I could think was, *I want to go home. This is all too real for me. Is this really happening?* Then I said, *Concentrate, we are here to get Lauren better. This is where she needs to be.* Thankfully, the room was private, and although not luxurious, it had a green vinyl couch and a reclining chair so at least Dean and I felt comfortable knowing we had places to sleep. After what seemed like hours, Lauren was finally comfortable in her bed, albeit with IVs and probes attached to her, connected to multiple monitors.

Over the next few days, there was a deluge of paperwork: consent forms to be signed and a health proxy among them. Signing the proxy, Dean signed as Lauren's alternate and we both hoped we'd never have to refer to it.

During the first week, Lauren was responding well to the treatment. Her fluid levels were going down and she was starting to feel better. I remember saying, "this is the longest doctor's appointment ever."

Chapter 4

Diary of Our Transplant Journey Begins

During our hospital stay, we found it very difficult to try to keep family and friends informed on Lauren's condition, having to repeat it all to everyone. Just being there was so exhausting; new worries and new procedures coupled with lack of sleep. The phone would ring and I would just look at it, knowing I couldn't talk without crying, so I wouldn't answer at all. I felt bad knowing others were concerned about Lauren too. Dean ended up being the one that would return calls for me during that time.

At that point, not knowing how long we were going to be in the hospital, I came up with what I thought was a great way to communicate with everyone…an online journal. Brilliant.

Looking around online, I was able to find a site allowing you to design your own journal format and style. Lauren and I found this was a great project for us to do together; it helped pass the time and allowed us to stay in touch with everyone through posts and messages back and forth. Discovering that most of these sites are free, it was perfect. If it's free, it's for us.

Chapter 5

Friday January 25, 2013

This is the journey of a young woman, my daughter, Lauren Meizo, in her fight for a new life. Lauren is a very brave, strong young woman. With everything she's endured, Lauren kept a positive attitude during this very difficult time. Lauren's signature word is ***STRENGTH*** and she has proven she has the strength to keep going.

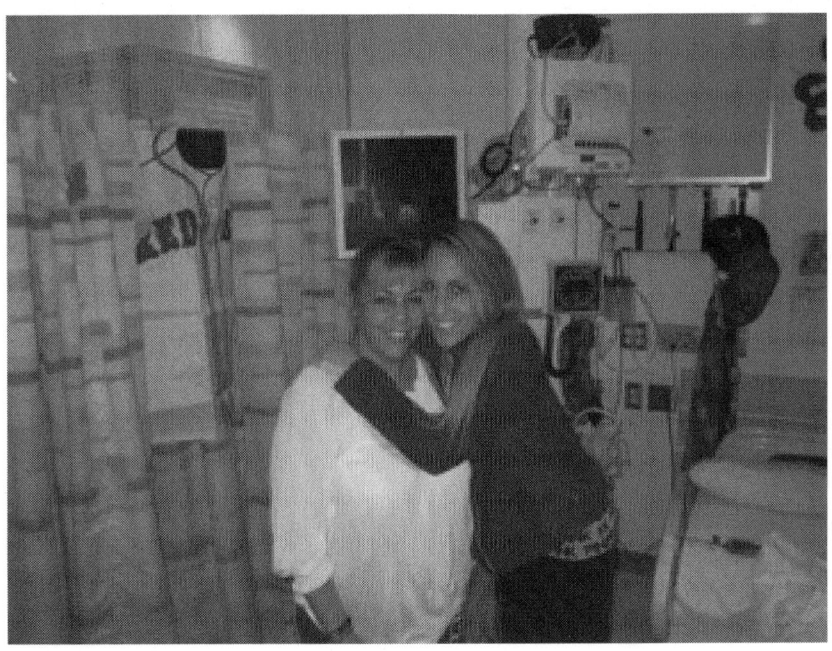

First entry: I decided to start a journal about my daughter Lauren, because at this point, it is very hard to talk on the phone to return calls. My daughter has many friends and family members that love her so much, so I realized this would be the best way to communicate with everyone and Lauren would be able to read comments that are sent to her.

This is my first general post and I will, down the road, fill in medical conditions, emotions, and overall well-being; both hers and mine. When a family member is sick, it's the whole family that feels it and the overwhelming feeling is one of helplessness.

Lauren's motto is "STRENGTH" so look for this word; it has many meanings but at this point, STRENGTH is what is going to take to help us remain both physically and emotionally strong.
Feel free to leave comments and words of encouragement.

Love, Lynne (Lauren's mom)

Saturday, January 26, 2013

Well, today is Day 10 in the hospital. We came here for a doctor's appointment to meet with a specialist; one who specializes in heart failure. After meeting with her, they admitted Lauren because she was in heart failure and the first step was to drain the fluids that were building up in her body. To date, she has lost 18 lbs., mostly fluids. (I have to say this is definitely the longest doctor's appointment we've ever had.)

At this point, her spirits are so-so, but I do have to say she has read all the comments this morning and she had a big smile on her face. Thanks everyone, it was great to see her smile.

This past Wednesday, Lauren had what's called a Pulmonary Artery (PA) catheter inserted into her neck; this allows the doctors to measure blood pressure and blood flow in the lungs and heart chambers. They took it out two days ago and it gave them the information they needed. We were told that next Wednesday they will have a plan to present to us. The doctors are talking about a mechanical heart pump or a heart transplant.

We have already started the Evaluation Process with the Multidisplinary Transplant Team. This group of highly skilled professionals is the one that decides if you would be approved to be on a transplant list.

To be placed on a list, it's a process; you have to be approved. A person may need a new organ but there could be reasons that they may not be placed on the list. The transplant team consists of a cardiologist, a cardiac transplant surgeon, nurse practitioners, a social worker, a psychiatrist, a nutritionalist, and a financial coordinator.

Along with Lauren being evaluated for approval, they had to evaluate Dean and myself as well. They needed to verify that we were up-to-date with all medical exams and we needed to show proof of all vaccinations. We also needed to show them pictures of our house; they needed to see what kind of environment Lauren lives in because her immune system would be compromised afterwards. We also needed to talk with social workers who want to make sure Lauren had a support system. So much is involved before you can even be approved to be listed. It's not an easy process.

Today they are doing a CAT scan on her lungs. She had a Cardiopulmonary Exercise Test done yesterday so they want to have a closer look. When they say "Transplant Team," they mean it. So many people are involved. I was having a hard time trying to remember names so Lauren and I would come up with nicknames. One doctor in particular came in wearing a beautiful pair of boots, so her nickname to us was "Boots." She got a kick out of it. Humor helps, no matter how bad it is.

I hope this has been helpful to all. I am trying my best to keep everyone informed. My hands are shaking as I'm typing (I hope this has spellcheck.) Lauren told me she will type a message to all later. I need to keep her motivated. Again thanks for all the well wishes, STRENGTH will get us through this. Love, Lynne

DAY OF REST

Monday, January 28, 2013

Hello all,

Today Lauren has a day of rest, NO TESTS. We had a very nice surprise from some wonderful friends from back home. Steve, Donna, Paul, Joe, Steph and Mark came to visit. It really made Lauren's day. Thank you guys so much for making the trip out here, you're the best.

Now get this one…

My mouth has been hurting me for the past few days and you would think being at the hospital 24/7, I could get a doctor to just take a quick peek…nope… not the case. It was like a bubble on my gum. Very painful, I just kept thinking stress was doing me in. The other night we had one of Lauren's favorite nurses on duty. Lauren said she was going to say something to her. I told her no; I was afraid that if I had something wrong with me they would have me leave her room. Well, Lauren told her. Long story short, I ended up in the emergency room!

The nurse called the ER, told them of my condition, and they told her send me down. When I arrived they were waiting for me. I do have to say I felt a little special being able to just walk right in. Turns out, giving in to my stubborn Polish ways, this time it paid off. I was told if I'd waited longer, I could be in real trouble. Without getting into details, I have an abscess. They sliced it, drained it, and wrote me a script. I feel 110% better.

Now a quick note from Lauren:

Hi, everyone! I just wanted to say thank you for the comments you've left and even those who just took the time to read about me. I didn't realize how truly sick I am until this experience. I haven't fully comprehended the idea that "hey, you may be a possible candidate for a HEART TRANSPLANT," but I'm sure it'll happen soon. Anyway, I just wanted to thank everyone for their support, and oh yeah, if you tried to text since the 16th (admission day) I've had my phone off. I'm not ignoring you, just have been so overwhelmed here. GAWWWW ! I love you all & when you start your day on Wednesday….just say a quick prayer for me <3

Love, Lynne & Lauren

Good Morning

Tuesday, January 29, 2013

This is Day 13 of "the longest doctor's appointment." With my infection, I have been getting very tired. I was able to find a drug store to get my script filled just a couple of blocks from the hospital and the walk felt good.

Lauren is off to her dentist appointment now. Yup, even her teeth need to be checked to make sure there are no cavities or any oral infections. I will give an update later on today. Need to get my thoughts together. Keeping spirits high. Love everyone for all your support for Lauren. God blessed her with great friends and family.

Wednesday, January 30, 2013

Good Evening,
I am tired of being here. With that said, I know Lauren feels the same, but worse, because she is one that has to undergo all the tests. I have it easy; my poor daughter has gone through the wringer. She is one tough cookie. I am very proud of her. With everything she is going through she worries about me. I tell her "we just need to take care of each other then one day we will go on vacation and really live it up."

The doctors told us that we might go home tomorrow. All tests have been concluded and Lauren has been stable. In my heart, once we go home, I know we will be returning but to go home for just a bit will be a slice of Heaven.

Lauren is getting stronger every day and now and then I will catch a smile on her face. She had a dental appointment today; they check everything here; she's going to need to get her wisdom teeth out. Other than that, she has a beautiful smile. I want to end this by saying thank you for all the STRENGTH everyone is sending her way.

Love, Lynne & Lauren

Chapter 6

We Are Home !!!!

Thursday, January 31, 2013

This is going to be a quick post.

Very, very tired; long day. We are finally home; that is the important thing at this time. I really discovered I'm not a city girl; hated it. I'm beat at this point and Lauren went to bed, so tomorrow I will fill everyone in on her condition and what the road ahead will look like.

Again, thanks for
all concerns.
We love you all,
Love, Lynne & Lauren

First Full Day Home

Thursday, January 31, 2013

Hello everyone,
I know I wanted to go into more detail about Lauren but at this point I am so burnt out. Today I had a ton of calls to make; insurance stuff.

We were both totally exhausted. She is doing well. That's all I have for today. Need to get more energy…….
Love, Lynne & Lauren

New Beginnings & Lifestyle Changes
Friday, February 1, 2013

Good Morning,
OK, I have a few minutes to myself this morning. I will try to sum up Lauren's condition. Yes, her heart has gotten weaker; it is working harder pumping the blood and the valve that has the leak doesn't help. They put her through every test out there during our stay in the hospital. Her body was retaining fluids (that is what happens when she goes into serious heart failure.) She lost 18 lbs. of fluid in the hospital. I know everyone is asking "Is she going to have a heart transplant?" Well, the answer is, only God knows at this time. She has a team of doctors that are wonderful. Very caring. Right now her body is too weak and she has a couple of more tests to do. More trips to Boston…..I will just sum it up as "yes, it could be on the plate but as far as when, let's just pray, 'never.'"

Now I am looking for help. Lauren is on a NO SODIUM diet. Sodium is like a sponge in her body (all of ours as well) and it holds extra fluid in the blood and body tissues. This extra fluid creates more work for the heart. Her diet allows her to have only 2000mg for the entire day. You might be thinking, "well, that doesn't sound so bad." Well it is. A normal person probably takes in around 5000-6000mg. Just as an example, a meal at McDonald's is around 3000mg, just in that one meal.

Last night my husband and I went grocery shopping. It took us two hours… We read every label on everything we bought. The sodium contents are staggering. Lauren is also on a fluid restriction, allowed only 64 ounces a day. Now this is not only liquids, this includes fruits that have water content!

So the goal is to keep fluids levels down and calorie intake up. Need to get some meat on those bones. To help her with this, my husband Dean and I are changing our diet so that she is not in this alone.

So I need some help…..If anyone has any good non-sodium or low-sodium recipes, please, please pass them on. She loves BBQ sauce but it is a no-no. Any ideas?

I hope this answers some questions you may have had. It is hard to think of everything. Also, I just wanted to pass on to everyone that if you leave a comment and you don't want it posted, let me know. Sometimes someone may want to leave a message for Lauren's eyes only.

Lots of Love,

Lynne & Lauren
(Pass on recipes, please)

New Week

Wednesday, February 6, 2013

Sorry I haven't updated in quite a few days, tired and a little busy. Lauren is doing well. Life adjustments are going on (diet the big one) for her and the family. I NEVER realized the sodium contents in food before, unbelievable.

At this point, just trying to get some weight on her and she is doing well. I want to thank everyone for the suggestions on recipes. I also found a couple of great websites on healthy heart eating.

My sister Donna drove up from Virginia to help me. I was feeling very overwhelmed and to be honest, couldn't think straight at times. To help me get organized, she put together a binder for all of Lauren's medical papers. Each folder in the binder is color-coded with tabs. Trust me, that book is becoming my bible. A folder for insurance papers, consent forms, list of medications and so on.

Donna is so great at helping us get everything organized. (She should go into business for herself as an organizer.) I really would not have been able to handle this all on my own. Just having her by our side is consoling.

Tomorrow, back to Boston. Not ready, but we need to do what we have to do. We are seeing Lauren's pulmonary specialist; they need to conduct tests on her lungs. This is another test to see if Lauren would qualify be become a candidate for a heart transplant. Send good thoughts our way…

Love,
Lynne & Lauren

Tuesday, February 12, 2013

Hello Everyone,

Time to update…..

On February 7th we went to back to Boston. Lauren had breathing tests done with her pulmonologist another doctor on her team. She needs everyone to be totally in agreement that Lauren could be accepted to be on the transplant list. This appointment is very important. (I know they all are) but the tests are going to tell us how Lauren's lungs are functioning. With her scoliosis, it puts more pressure on her lungs. Well, with that being said, it was a good appointment. FINALLY some good news. So if and when Lauren needs, she would be able to have a heart transplant. **So the window of opportunity is open.** We can move forward with treatment plans for her.

On a lighter note, my sister Donna came with us. I do not know if you know about the city of Boston but for a country girl like me, I hate driving in the city. You can get lost so fast. Well, it was very confusing to find the hospital and yes, we did have our GPS. We left the doctor's at 4pm and got home at 8:30pm. It took us one hour just to get out of the parking garage! Then we got lost and stuck in traffic, so needless to say, my sister, who travels a lot, saw most of the city. At one point she said, "Hey, there's Boston Garden." The hospital was nowhere *near* there.

This past Monday we were supposed to go back to Boston to meet with our Nurse Practitioner Heart Failure/Transplant Cardiovascular Division at Brigham and Women's Hospital. With the weather calling for ice, we did a phone meeting. Not the same, but still, we were able to discuss Lauren's weight and medications. She is our go-to person with any types of questions we may have, plus support. At this point, we have appointments every week in Boston. They are keeping a close eye on her. It's a scary feeling knowing that your daughter is sick. I can say that during the night I get up a couple of times just to check on her Lauren is feeling good, gaining weight and getting rest. With her NO SALT diet, that is the way I cook now. I do have to say my own weight, as well as Dean's, is going down from eating just healthy, no-sodium food. (Or just stressed.) Still working on so much paper work. Lauren's on a leave of absence from work and school is on hold. So to any of her friends around the area, please stop by. Annette, whenever you are ready to start painting, let us know. Lauren wants to make-over her bedroom.

A sad day is approaching: my sister Donna is leaving to go back home to Virginia on Saturday. I love her so much for all the help and support she gives me and my whole family. Love you, sis !!!!!

Love,
Lynne & Lauren

Monday, February 18, 2013

On today's post I just want to say a big THANK YOU to everyone who has sent prayers and good thoughts our way. Lauren has been feeling good. She is now in the process of re-doing her bedroom with a wonderful friend, Annette. She needs this to keep her busy and excited. Thank you, Annette, for taking the time to do this with her.

Last Friday I bought a new car. It was Valentine's Day. 2010 Honda Accord 3.5 ELX Coupe. My husband met me at the dealership and said "If this is the car you want, let's get it." We traded-in the Mountaineer so now I have a beautiful smaller car to make all our rides to Boston. Great Valentine's gift. Now I will be able to become a Boston driver; you know the type, you have to be able to zip in and out of traffic. No offense to Boston drivers but you need to know how to drive in a big city atmosphere. Love my new car.

Love,
Lynne & Lauren

Back to Boston

Wednesday, February 20, 2013

Lauren has an appointment with her Heart Failure Specialist in Boston. The last time we had an appointment with her, she admitted Lauren for two weeks. So now we each have a bag packed, just in case.

I am really anxious to be going to this appointment; lately, Lauren has been having good days and not-so-good days. She makes me very nervous. I am just a bag of nerves at this point. Let's just hope we come home!

It's going to be our first trip in the new car; so glad I have it now.

I am working on trying to post pictures and as soon as I figure it out I have some good ones to post.

Love,
Lynne & Lauren

We're Home!
Thursday, February 21, 2013

Hey Everyone, This is Lauren

So I decided to take the laptop from Mom and write today's post….

I'll start with how today went seeing my Heart Failure Specialist (the doctor that admitted me initially)…

This time mom and I went prepared. I had my bag with a bunch of different outfits so I didn't wear the same outfits over and over again & my make-up, movies, bath products, etc… JUST IN CASE, and mom did the same. Over the past few days I haven't felt the greatest to the point I honestly thought I was going to be admitted again. I was feeling the same symptoms I had last time…shortness of breath, very tired to the point I barely was out of bed, felt like I was going to throw up, wicked horrible stomach pains (almost like someone kept punching me over & over again-I felt the last time and I thought it was just a bug, but turned out to be basically all my belly organs swollen from fluids), and lastly, I've gained weight.

Now down to business - How'd the appointment go?
Well, after the exam the doctor decided to NOT admit me! YAY !! But she did change around my medications. She took me off two of them for a short period of time to see if my blood pressure will increase and as for my "pee pills," they were increased since my initial discharge

from 20mg is now up to 80mg. Make sense? You are probably asking, "what is the plan for the transplant?" Well…the doctor brought it up and the way she worded it - it won't be in 20 years or 10 years or 5 years…rather, sooner. Ugh! So basically at this point we're just letting my current heart work until it can't pump anymore… then transplant. My doctor made sure to stress the fact that I have very severe heart disease. She didn't admit me because I really haven't gained enough fluids or looked like a balloon like the last time. So, to wrap this appointment up…I had blood work done and will be returning in exactly two weeks to see how I have been doing. At this point in time, I am actually gaining real weight with some extra fluid in there.

I want to thank everyone for their thoughts and prayers and keeping my family and I in mind. It means a lot, more than you could ever imagine. By the way, I'm going to start doing more writing so everyone knows how "Lauren" feels about everything.

I want to thank my mom for starting this journal; now I feel strong enough to write with her. I am feeling all the love and the STRENGTH to battle this. Love everyone and thank you for keeping me in your prayers. It really means so much to me….

Tuesday, February 26, 2013

This is the first week we do not have to go to Boston. Lauren has been feeling good and has been getting stronger. One day at a time. My sister sent me some great cookbooks on no-sodium recipes. Doing so much studying on how important your diet is has really opened my eyes. It's time to get Lauren back to the gym; she really used to love going, so we're getting her butt there this week. Baby steps….. the doctors told me it would be good for her to build up her strength. If she will need a transplant, it is so important that she is as strong as she can be.

Gym Day

Thursday, February 28, 2013

Today Lauren and I went to the gym. It makes me so nervous for her to go but she needs to keep her muscles strong. We went on the treadmill and I kept having her check her heart rate. I had to keep telling her to slow down. Then we did some lifting; I was putting very light weights on for her and she was like "Really, Mom?!" I told her: baby steps. We had a great time.

As far as her diet is concerned, she is doing a great job following it. She is putting on weight, but very, very slowly. She is on a high-calorie, no sodium diet and I am on a low-calorie, no sodium diet.

Next week it's back to Boston, Monday then Wednesday. Thank God for the new car, great on gas.
Love,
Lynne & Lauren

Back to Boston Tomorrow
Monday, March 4, 2013

On the road again.
Tomorrow we have two appointments in Boston. First appointment is with the surgeon that implanted her defibrillator last year. She had that surgery March 15, 2012; this visit is just a check-up.

Then we have an appointment with a nutritionist. I am really excited about this appointment to learn more about Lauren's diet. Diet is so important in her health and I have been doing so much studying so I have many questions to ask a professional. It's going to be a busy day. Lauren has been trying to be as active as her body will allow. We have been going to the gym a lot and I have to say, she is tough. I make sure she doesn't overdo it too much but on the other hand, she pushes me like crazy. I call her my little spider monkey. The other day, we were working on abs and at one point I said I had to stop because I was getting a cramp and Lauren said "o bad, give me two more." So I did. She is my Jillian Michaels (from "The Biggest Loser"). Love this kid.

Chapter 7

Here We Go Again

They say life is filled with surprises. We try to think we are prepared for anything that may be thrown at us. Growing up, you have to overcome many obstacles that will prepare you for life. Living life, I've found out the hard way to never take anything for granted. Life is a gift. Life is not forever. Life is always changing.

Friday, March 8, 2013

This is Donna, Lynne's sister.

She asked me to update…

Lauren wasn't felling well. After calling the doctor, they told Lynne they wanted to see Lauren. So on Wednesday they headed back to Boston. I am sad to report that they admitted Lauren. Her fluid levels around her heart were way up. The family is camped out in Room 927. Lynne and Lauren had the trunk packed, just in case she was to be admitted. Lynne even has her own coffee pot. I was told the nurses said her room smelled amazing and Lynne informed them she was going to bake cookies next, of course, after she straightened up the room and cleaned the floor, LOL.

Lauren is doing okay. Bored, wants to go home, so send her all your STRENGTH and prayers. Visitors are welcome and snacks too (low-sodium of course.) Lynne will post an update as soon as the doctors discuss what comes next.

Thanks,

Donna

CHAPTER 8

THE DECISION HAS BEEN MADE LAUREN IS ON THE HEART TRANSPLANT LIST

LIFE AS WE KNOW IT WILL NEVER BE THE SAME

Wednesday March 13, 2013

It's been a week now since we've been in the hospital and I haven't been able to even open up the computer. I want to thank my sister Donna for helping keep everyone informed. Thanks, sis.

Ok here it is: Lauren is now on the heart transplant list. The transplant team walked into Lauren's room and told us she was approved to be placed on the list. APPROVED. Now our journey really begins. To be approved means Lauren could have a second chance at life. It means there is hope for my daughter. Not everyone is accepted to be placed on a transplant list, for many reasons. We have been blessed.

Lauren is today at a 1-B static. Tomorrow she will be in a 1-A static. What that means is she is high priority, top of the list. Her blood type is B, which is not common. When I say that tomorrow she will be a 1-A is because she is going to have a procedure called a Pulmonary

Artery Catheter injected into to neck. She will have this line in her neck until the transplant. Every ten days they will have to take it out and redo the procedure, to change the spot and check to make sure no infection sets in. On that one day, it will give her a little relief. (My poor child.) So at this point, this means she will be bed-bound. The catheter line is only so long and it will be hooked up to medications that are connected to many machines. My heart is totally breaking. I wish God would have me go through this, not my daughter.

At Brigham & Women's Hospital last year they did sixteen heart transplants, all successful. What we found out is, the data base for organs is in Virginia. It is called UNOS, United Network for Organ Sharing. Now WHEN they have a heart for Lauren, they have a four hour window to get it to her. So we are going to be staying in the hospital until she receives her new heart. When that will be, only the Dear Lord knows. Days, weeks, months, years.

I am living here with Lauren; she is very scared (so am I). My husband's life is a living hell as well. During the week, he is home so he can go to work, then on Fridays he drives to Boston straight from work to spend the weekend with us. He has the lovely privilege of sleeping in a recliner. Then on Sunday he drives home.

Again, thanks for all the prayers and well wishes. I think I summed up everything but I am sure I forgot a lot. In my heart I do not know why such a beautiful and caring person would have to go through this.

Thursday, March 14, 2013

This is Donna again, received a phone call from Dean this morning. Lauren is trying to stay positive. Scared, too many emotions. She wants her life back. To help keep her spirits up, Lauren wants to spruce up her room. She said she needs to dazzle and decorate her room because we don't know how long she will be waiting for her new heart.

Keep sending your prayers and if you get a chance, go visit the family camped out in Room 927. Bring something dazzling for her room.

Thanks,
Donna

Day 19, On My Way To A New Life
Sunday March 24, 201

Hi everyone,

This is Lauren actually posting for once. Sorry for the lack of posts, we'll be updating more often. Things have just been crazy. So here's a brief update before I share how I actually feel…

Yes, I was finally placed on the heart transplant list on March 13th, as my mom had previously told you. I need to have a "PA line" in my neck with two special medicines helping my heart beat stronger to be considered a 1A, top of the list.

Well, I ended up getting the line in on that Friday and things were looking great until about 10:30 at night. My mom was rubbing my feet, trying to relax me so I could fall asleep, when all of a sudden my heart rate started going up. Long story short, ordeal went on until almost 2am. My room was filled with doctors and nurses form the ICU. One of the doctors tried to jiggle the line. Once he had done that, all hell broke loose. I think there was a kink or something because after that a ton of the medicine released and my heart rate went up to 158. I had an x-ray machine in my room, EKGs done, the whole nine yards. My mom was crying because you can literally see my heart beating through my 101 lb. body. All of a sudden, my nurse told me they were ready to sedate me….and put the shock stickers on me. Yup, they were ready to jolt my ass. Scary!! Instead, they ended up pulling the line and for the rest of the weekend I was bumped down to a 1B status.

It was a stressful weekend because we were unsure if I was going to be able to get the "LEASH" (PA line) back in my neck. I call it a leash as a joke because I only have about a three foot radius to walk around with it in….. just imagine being twenty-two years old and basically being bed bound for ten days at a time while all your friends are progressing and having fun with their lives. Actually, imagine being *any* age and told you have to deal with this.

On Monday, it went back in on the other side of my neck and so far, things have been looking good from that standpoint, but I must admit, I freakin' hate it. My Auntie Donna came all the way from Virginia to spend the week at the hospital with Mom and I. You see, my dad, (I call him Fosha) had to go home to go to work. On Fridays, when he gets out of work, he hits the road to spend the weekend with us. Well, my Aunt did not come empty-handed. She ended up decorating my room with things that people have been bringing me. I must admit,everyone says I have the best looking room on the floor. So if you come visit or send something, make sure it's colorful, hint-hint, wink-wink. With my aunt being here, my heart failure specialist told my mom to go home for a day and take it all in because I'm going to need her sane (LOL) for the long haul. I love you, Auntie Donna. She had me smiling and laughing the whole time although Mom said she felt horrible being away from me.

So how do I feel about all this?

Hmmmm…today I was told that their best guess is most likely like late spring/early summer; not weeks, but months. This isn't fair, although I've made friends with pretty much everyone I've met. I wish I wasn't here. I feel trapped and overwhelmed. When I first found out the news, I felt selfish and guilty. Why, you may ask yourself? Because I'm literally sitting here and praying for someone to die just so I can have a second chance at life. But as the doctors and others have explained….it's not like you killed them. I will have nothing to do with their death; what is meant to be, is meant to be. They also said that the victim's families often find peace knowing that their loved one was able to go on and help someone else to live. Therefore, now I feel a bit better about that topic.

Next post: tomorrow…

I just don't want this post to be ten pages long and honestly, my thoughts are everywhere. I will try to update every day because I need a way to release my stress and actually share with you in-depth rather than just an "okay."

It's 11:30pm right now and rounds and blood draws are at six in the morning so I'm going to end this one for tonight and pick it back up tomorrow.

Like always, I want to thank everyone for their prayers, gifts, and visits. It's helping me chug through this so please keep it all coming. I know Boston isn't close, but I can have visitors and do enjoy seeing loving faces.

OH YEAHHHH.. Mom, Auntie Donna and I are going to be setting up an online fundraiser to help with medical bills and all the prescriptions I'll be adding to my already mile-long list and everything else this adventure brings. So please continue to check the journal for updates. Honestly, any little bit helps.

Thank you for letting me ramble and I know I missed so many things I am just going to end this with…as smiling and optimistic and cheerful as you know me as.. I would never wish what I am going through on my worst enemy; sometimes I feel like I'm being punished for something.

Anyway, God bless and I love you all very much. I wouldn't be able to do this without your support, even the staff here has commented on the fact my room is always filled with visitors and I have
great support, so
thank you all.

Love always

Lauren

Lauren Unleashed
Thursday, March 28,2013

Hi there,

Sorry it's been a couple of days since I've posted, but like usual it's been busy and then by the time I'm free…my thoughts are either jumbled or I'm exhausted. So today was the tenth day of the "leash" (PA line in my neck.) Today I was able to walk around. I even went outside with my mom and a nurse for 5 minutes to breath in the fresh Boston air. I've learned in the past ten days of being basically bed bound, of all the little things I had taken for granted. Imagine wishing and wanting to just wash your hands under warm running water. I was. I only had buckets filled with warm water and soap to wash myself clean and to wash my hands after going to the bathroom. Yeah, that's right..that's how I showered. I won't take take the idea of showering for granted ever again. I felt like a prisoner set free. I mean, I was still hooked to a heart monitor and an IV poll with the medication helping keep my heart working a bit stronger, but at least I was able to get up and walk around.

So since I have the line out, I dropped from a 1A to a 1B which pulls me off from the top priority, but tomorrow I will have the line put right back in and it's back to losing my freedom for another 10 days. They go a cycle of 10 days, in case you were wondering, to avoid infection if left in longer and to try and cause the least amount of trauma. So they have found a fair balance with that time frame.

Now I'm going to leave this post 'to be continued..' I'm tired from all the running around I did today.. hah !! And I need my beauty rest plus a good nights sleep for tomorrow's procedure. To have the PA line put back in I have to go to the Cath Lab. It's a scary ordeal, it is done in an operating room. Sterile environment. I promise I'll get more in depth and share more of the bullshit I have been living through. Also I just wanted to throw out there again…a fundraiser is in the works to help my family and I. It is going to be online, so I will post the link when it's all set. I would like to just try and start my second chance at life with the least amount of stress from this ordeal as possible.

Next time you wash your hands, take a shower, or step outside and take a deep breath of fresh air…think of me and remember those small things are what I'm fighting for my life to do.

Love,

Lauren

I Used to Like Rollercoaster Rides....

Wednesday, April 3, 2013

Growing up I used to get excited about riding the big, tall, scary rollercoaster…but I must say this rollercoaster ride isn't as fun with its ups and downs.

I apologize for not posting in a few days…it all finally sunk in. To be honest, I've been in a funk. I love everyone's support and cards and flowers and such but I don't want to be here anymore. Don't get me wrong, I love visitors!! So please keep coming. It kills me inside when they go to leave and I can't walk out with them. I feel like a prisoner. I had no idea in a million years that when you were listed for a transplant that this is how you were going to live your "waiting time," tied up.

Those that know me best would think that I should be in my glory..getting to stay in bed all day and sleep, but to tell you the truth, after all this, I don't want to see another damn bed for the rest of my life. Prior to all this I was active. I had a life, a job, I was going to school. and going out with friends but that all changed March 16th when I was admitted. I realize I need to focus on the future, on the prize..a new heart is-pretty much a second chance at life. This is by far is the hardest thing I've ever had to do. If you think about it, even if I got a heart and went into surgery at this second, I still have a good month's worth of hospital stay, minimum! Yeah, that's right, I'm going to bitch and complain in this post because this is how I feel. This is my experience.

I can't always be upbeat and smiling. I'm too young for this. Everyone else on the floor is much, much older. I was playing chess with an 80-year-old man the other day when I had my leash off!! The worst part is, I have no idea when this nightmare is going to be over. Once I get a new heart, it's going be a completely new lifestyle. I'll be on multiple medications due to my immune system being greatly compromised for the rest of my life (that's the reason for the fundraiser..they're expensive).

Ever since I was ten, it's felt like while my friends went to play, I just felt different because no one else I knew was going through this. I know they say God only gives you what you can handle. Well, if that is true then God thinks I'm invincible!! I need a break, I wish I could take a vacation from myself. Like I said, I apologize for rambling and complaining but at this point this is the only way I feel like I can release some stress without putting it on my parents. Day in and day out, I have to watch my mother and see how much this is killing her to watch her baby girl going through this and all she can do is get me my tooth brush and a cup of water or a drink or grab my crayons so I can color. It eats at me, to be honest, I feel guilty. This isn't how I want her spending her life. See, I'm sitting here waiting for a freakin' heart transplant and I'm more worried about my mother's well-being and sanity.

This is basically how a day goes for me… at 6am I usually get woken up to have my blood drawn. Then shortly after the intern doctor examines me. From there I receive all 17 out of 18 morning pills, yum. I have my vitals done and I'm weighed daily (after I pee to get rid of any extra fluids in me). Then the transplant team come in. The attending top doctor and the fellow examine me as well. My room has about 8 to 9 people in here at once. The clock hasn't even reached 9am yet. Gotta eat breakfast since I'm on a strict diet. Might I also add, every hour my nurse needs to come in and print a PA line strip to do measurements from my catheter in my neck, love this so they use a painter's leveler to level the machine to my heart (ANNOYING). Lunch comes usually followed by or given with 4-5 more meds. I usually take a nap after that because I'm tired from all the wonderful festivities. When I wake up I try to do something to take my mind away from everything that is going on. I think I am the best colorer ever by now.. haha. Don't get me wrong, I have plenty of things to keep me busy.

I was attending college in Boston, so I have made many friends that live close by. My friend Breen has been visiting so frequently that that I would be lost without you. Anyways…night time always consists of another blood draw (my arms and hands have so many poke holes and black and blues..if you didn't know my situation you'd think I was a druggie- it's horrible), more nighttime meds depending on what my blood lab report shows and we can't forget my nightly shot of Lovanox. Lovanox is a shot that has to be given in my stomach; it's a blood thinner and since I'm in a bed all day it helps prevent blood clots. It hurts a lot..stings. It's notorious for the pain. Mind you, throughout the day my vitals are taken and then there are the various extras such as EKGs, IV tubing lines being changed, chest rays, catheter changes and so on and so on.

Some might think that just being in bed all day doesn't sound like anything to bitch about but when it's going on a month and you feel like a puppet doing what the doctors and nurses tell me to do, it's horrible. I'm blessed that I do have this chance at a second life and I really shouldn't complain about that, but c'mon!! I'm too young for this. Seeing my friends having lives really does kill me and I'll admit something that I never thought I'd admit to all…but I'm jealous. I have to have my ribcage latterly sawed open and to put it bluntly, not have a heart in my body for a short period of time, while others will never have to fathom that idea. It is a rollercoaster ride. I worry. I worry about myself, my parents and what this is doing to my loved ones. I worry about the financial burden this is and will put me through.

GRRRRRR! I feel a bit better for venting. I really need to stick to updating this all more often. Keeping it bottled up for a couple of days makes me end up like that. All I can ask is that everyone continue to pray for myself and my family.

I'm learning you do have your ups and downs of emotions during this process like a rollercoaster. I know I can get through this and I am strong enough, it just going to be a long ride, so looks like we all need to hold on tight

.

Chapter 9

One Month In and Counting

Thursday April 11, 2013

I'm beginning to realize I suck at updating. My apologies, but to be honest, it's like I'm stuck in limbo waiting here. I just recently "cele-brated" my one-month anniversary here. And to think this all started out as a doctor's appointment; we expected to be home by 1pm that day. But as we all know, that was not the case. Some days are rougher than others like I previously mentioned but I'm trying to keep a smile on my face as big as I can. Every day seems to feel like Groundhog's Day here; the same old, same old for the most part. I feel like my life is on pause. Everyone else I know is moving forward and I'm stuck in bed except on the tenth day of the line, then the leash gets to come out and I get to shower and sit on the couch instead of my bed. I usually walk the halls and talk with EVERYONE in sight. Not to toot my own horn or anything but they all love me here, LOL. I know they love my room; every day I acquire more and more flowers and wall hangings. I love it!!! My room looks like a dorm room, as the nurses and doctors call it. Some have even commented that my room looks better than their apartments.

I think it's time to blow this popsicle stand. I want to go home. The other day the line was supposed to come out on Saturday but I request-ed to be leashed up an extra day until Sunday. You may ask yourself, after all the bitching I do about it, why would I want to keep it in an extra day? Reason being: the cath lab only runs Monday-Friday except for emergencies. By keeping the PA line in, it is giving me an extra day as a top priority 1A. Had I had it out on Saturday, then I'd be a 1B, less of priority.

So Monday I went down to get it back in and even with the amount of sedation equal to that for a horse, I still found myself crying. I apparently have a tiny blood clot and it redirected the line and hit a nerve TWICE!! The pain was unbearable. I started crying and shaking to the point I had to ask the "bartender" for more cocktails (the nurse for more Fentanyl). The doctor had to call in another doctor to help position it apparently. I don't know, I couldn't see with all the drapes over my face. A one-hour procedure from leaving my room to returning, took close to four hours. Mom was pacing and crying, worrying because it had taken so long, poor thing.

The rest of the day the PA line tracing looked good. Early Tuesday morning it started to dampen-out and not look so great. The attending doctor came in early that morning and played with the line because it was in a wedge, which means too close to my lungs. Everything went well for a short period of time, then the line apparently ended up in my right ventricle, which according to my nurse, if not taken out can be very, very dangerous. So I was irritated and sore because I was afraid the line was going to have to come out. The doctors had to keep playing with it, resulting in an x-ray to make sure the placement was right. I'll admit, the line in the neck, once the skin is healed around the tube, doesn't bother me as much, so that's a positive.

While in the hospital, I've learned a lot. Starting with the medical aspect, a few of my nurses have taught me how to do the math and figurations of the PA line strips as well as how to stop my IV drip machine from beeping without a nurse. (I usually get in trouble for this, LOL.)

Also, not to mention I've taken an interest in the court system. Every day I watch my "Judge Joe Brown," "the People's Court," then "Judge Judy".. ha ha. Seriously, I don't know where they find these people to go on these shows. I feel like an old lady…I HAVE to watch my programs every day. So out of this I can be a doctor/ nurse/lawyer.

This experience has brought me closer to family members and friends where relationships previously had either been broken or fuzzy. By the way, Mom and I would like to thank my mom's cousins, Kristen, Karen, and Auntie Ginger for the beautiful Alex & Ani heart bracelets…we put them on and vowed we'd both never take them off. They were sent with love.

Please visit me……

I miss my life. I want to go back to work. I want to finish school. I want to bust my ass at the gym, I want to snuggle, I want to breathe fresh air. I want to feel rain. I want to drive my car. I want to pet my dog, Ralfy. Basically, what I'm getting at is I have a new bucket list. But aside from the slump I've been in, God does everything for a reason and He knew I'd be able to handle this no matter how many blood draws I'd need, or neck cats, or the lifestyle changes to come. I'm known for my STRENGTH and ability to fight through any situation thrown my way, but more importantly, I couldn't do this without all of you.

P.S. - My mom has spent 99% of the time at the hospital and has decided to crochet me a blanket with different color yarns that friends have given us so I always have it to remember for the rest of my life. Point is, if you'd like to send a roll of yarn, any color you choose, she'll add it in and please include a short note why you chose that color, this way I'll think of you every time I look at it or curl up with it. Thank you.

Please keep my family in your prayers, like you have been, and don't be afraid to ask if you'd like to visit. Also, for all of you that use Facebook, if you wouldn't mind posting this site to spread the word. I would appreciate it more than you'd ever know.

Love to the
moon & back,
Lauren

Pulmonary Artery Catheter Line (PA line)
a/k/a Swan-Ganz Wedge verses RV

Friday, April 12, 2013

I would like to try to explain more about my PA line. The doctors are always checking to make sure the line isn't in wedge or RV. When you hear me talk about wedge verse RV, I don't mean I have a wedgie or motor vehicle, LOL. As you know and can see from the photo posted, I have a neck catheter that I have in for ten days on, and one day off. Well, the catheter line, when put in, is not completely secured to one spot; it can move toward the lungs and if left there long enough, it can cause bleeding and tissue damage. This is called "wedge."

RV is when the tip of the catheter is wiggling around in the right ventricle; this can cause fluttering of the heart and an irregular heartbeat. Since I have a defibrillator in me, it will then shock me. Also, if I'm in RV for an extended period of time, Ventricular Tachycardia can occur, with all that the blood flow being blocked and organs such as my brain, liver, and kidneys possibly suffering damage & eventually dying..

So to sum it up, wedge versus RV, are not good things at all. Obviously, there is more science to it and I didn't explain it as well as a medical professional would have, but that's just the best way I could explain it in my own words.

Last night the doctors were in my room for over an hour just getting my PA line back to where it safely needs to be for the accurate readings they need. The fellow doctor, the one under the top dog, left me at 11pm and was called back into the hospital at about 1am and stayed until 2:45am, just to be back here again at 7am for his shift. In that time, I had a chest x-ray done. Once Dr. Ben left, the doctor from the CCU (ICU) took over to try and get me in a safe spot. I had to sleep in one position the whole night because the slightest move could've send me either into wedge or RV, while a nurse sat directly outside my room watching the monitor all night.

Today has been nothing but a pain in the neck, no pun intended. As I type this, the line is still giving me trouble. I'm praying that they don't remove the line since it's Friday and the cath lab only does this Monday-Friday. If they take the line out today or tomorrow, that means I'd be dropped down to a 1B lower status for a longer period of time. To you, one or two days may not seem like it's be a problem or make any difference, but those one or two days could be "that moment" I've been waiting for. So truthfully, every second the catheter is in is one step closer to my new life.

Not to sound like a Debbie Downer or anything, but this experience is something I'd never imagine. I constantly have anxiety; yes, I'm on medication for it, because I never know when I'll get that call. Or there is the possibility that I'm asked if I want to be a back-up for someone, so I'm prepped, thinking this could be the big moment and the first person takes the heart. Or another scenario: I'm approached by the doctors but they tell me it is considered a "high risk" heart, meaning high risk of infection due to actions the donor had made in their lifetime. In this instance, I can decline that heart; I most likely would, just because I'm young and why would I want to go through all this for a shitty heart? If I choose to do that, I am not in trouble or penalized against being in the running for another heart because everyone on the list has a number.. .not their name given on it. Mentally, it is just draining and upsetting.

Day in and day out, you have no idea what could possibly happen. Hell, the doctors could walk right in now and say "Lauren, don't eat or drink anything." Only God knows when the day will come. To tell you the truth, I could never tell you how I feel or how scared I really am,. I think God and I socialize more now than when I was in Catholic school.

Please keep myself and my family in your thoughts and prayers. Even though my family members aren't the actual patients, this is taking an unbelievable emotional toll on them having to watch me suffer. I just want to live and continue on with my life like YOU are doing.

Oh!! Once again, on a happier note, if you see a scrap of yarn again, please send it with a note why that color so I'll always remember you in my blanket my mom is making. If you plan on visiting, please let us know ahead of time just in case it's not a good day, please.

Thank you for all your love

and support,

Lauren<3

Today is Day 44

A Mother's Love

Thursday, April 18,

2013

Hello all,

This is Lynne, Lauren's mom. This morning I got up and counted how many days Lauren and I have been here. It's 44 days and counting. It feels like a lifetime but I have to stay positive. This is only the beginning of our journey. As I sit here in our new home (for the time being) I look around in disbelief that we are here now. In the past 44 days, friends and family have come here to decorate the room to make it feel as comfortable as possible.

My son Mike brought Lauren an ultra-comfy mattress pad to make her bed super soft. My sister Donna brought me comfy bedding as well. My bed is a vinyl couch that looks like a day bed now. I even have a rug in front of my bed, thanks to Donna. One wall is covered with all the cards Lauren has received. She absolutely loves reading cards and letters. One day, they brought a U.S. Mail tote to the room because she had so many cards and gifts. I WANT TO SAY THANK YOU ALL, it really means a lot.

I have so many emotions going through me, I would like to share some of them. Years ago we found out that Lauren had medical problems, as we went from doctor's appointments and numerous hospitals. In my wildest dreams I never thought it would bring us to this point. I sit here and watch my daughter lying in bed with tubes and lines all connected to her; the major one in her neck. My heart just breaks. I am blessed that when she is awake, she is, for the most part, in good spirits. She loves to color and she's pretty good at staying inside the lines.

I have many, many thoughts that go through my head all the time. One being how very blessed we are that Lauren was accepted to be on the heart transplant list. One day she will receive the most important gift she can ever get: a heart. A start to a new life.

Okay, now I want to vent……..I need to get it out. The hospital has been great; physically and emotionally, with Lauren. Not complaining, but okay, maybe a little. It is so hard sitting here as a mother and waiting and watching everything that is going on with little support for me. There have been many days of crying (not in front of Lauren). Everyone here thinks I am so strong, but inside I am not. I have so much bottled up that every now and then I just break down. The last time was Sunday, and even today my eyes are still puffy and red. People have asked me who punched me in the eye. Every day I am on pins and needles saying *maybe today?*

At this point, I know only one person who can probably understand how I am feeling; two years ago her daughter went through the same thing. Her daughter had her heart transplant and I am so happy to say she is doing wonderfully. I find comfort communicating with her. Thank You.

I miss my home, my granddaughter, my husband, my son, my life. Living in the hospital is so hard. Big Brother is always watching. NO PRIVACY. People just walk in the room all the time. So many times I think, *I would love to put a lock on the inside, but I know that is a no-no.* I am not used to everyone knowing my business all the time. They do say I keep this room very tidy and clean.

44 days down, who knows…maybe

today.

Keep praying for us

Love,
Lynn

Chapter 11
Boston Marathon

My Life is on Pause

Boston is on Pause
Friday, April 19, 2013

Well, you don't need me to tell you how crazy of a week it's been, just turn on the TV and you can see it, but imagine being in THE hospital of interest or looking out the window seeing a SWAT team on the roof while police & the FBI guard every entrance with machine guns. Like I'm not stressed out enough as it is, nor is my family….now every hour or so we hear "Code Amber," meaning expect a large amount of people headed to the emergency room.

Marathon Monday, I remember watching TV while I was being prepped for my PA line procedure in the cath lab. It all went smoothly and when I returned to my room to get hooked up and situated, my nurse told me I had two male visitors. I didn't know who it could be; turned out it was my friend Sean and a friend of his. He had a card for me. He gave it to the nurse to give to me and I wanted to see him personally, since he came to visit me, so they hung around and waited. When I was done getting situated in my bed, I finally was able to visit with them. They stayed about 20 minutes or so as we took pictures, laughed, then hugged and kissed goodbye. They were headed down to watch the race at the finish line.

At 3:44pm I received a text from Sean…"*If I didn't wait to see you I would have been where the explosion happened. You are my guardian angel and I love you.*" I instantly cried, I had already known of the horrific details, since I was at one of the main hospitals…so I heard stuff that was happening. I texted my other buddy who'd spent the night with his cousin in B&WH ER, holding her hand. As he described it to me, she kept shouting "where's my leg!?" He described the ER scene just below me as a horrid war zone: people missing limbs, the smell of burning flesh. Unbelievable. I wish I could get into greater detail on certain topics but just know that even though the doors of the hospital are locked and guarded by cops with machine guns, I still have an uneasy feeling in my stomach.

My nurse wanted me to turn my TV off because watching the news was making me shake and shooting my heart rate upwards of 140 bpm so my screen was flashing red and making an obnoxious noise; this was even after my high dosage of Valium. It's completely scary knowing the bomb went off about a mile from the hospital.

So this was actually a question/ thought I had that made me feel heartless, no pun intended, but I looked at my mom and said "maybe I could get a heart from this." She said she didn't even think of that, so I thought I should ask the doctors and they said if they had to take a guess, no. And to be truly honest, if I was to be offered a heart right now, after what had happened on Monday…even though I'd have no idea where the heart came, I don't think I'd want to get my heart this

close to this current situation. Personally, it would just always draw me back to this memory and I do realize that either way, for me to continue my life, someone does have to sadly die but I don't want to be like this.
Tuesday they switched my pain meds but I was still in crazy pain. I kinda kept my mouth shut when I wasn't feeling well. I felt guilty, like, here I am with both legs and arms and no debris from the bomb and I'm complaining while people are being induced into comas to help control their pain. I felt greedy and I needed to keep telling myself, *Lauren, you're in the hospital for a heart transplant, not for a hangnail.* I actually felt so strongly about this, I needed to talk to a medical professional to be reassured to speak up if I'm in pain.

Update: pain meds were increased and I'm comfortable again.

Another thing I want to just briefly touch on: it is amazing that in both instances with the bombing, how everyone is coming together. I mean, even the Yankees sang "Sweet Caroline" in New York for Boston. Also, for me personally, the transplant pushed me to join Facebook again and I'm glad I did. The support I'm feeling from the site alone is unbelievable and like I put in a post before, one doctor told me: "One of the best ways to get through this, Lauren, is having a great support system" and I've learned this to be true. The amount of people I have supporting me is amazing. I didn't realize how much I meant to people

73

This is better than ADT Security

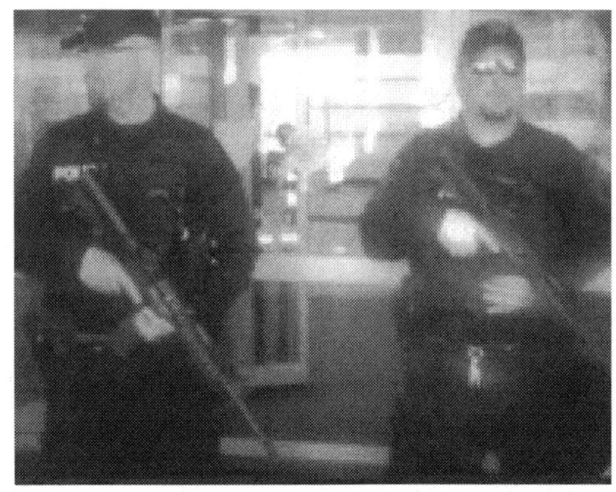

The hospital was on lockdown for quite a few days. When Mom went outside, she would have to show her ID to be able to enter the building again. Inside, on the main floor, there were armed guards everywhere. My mom said it "felt like a war zone." We've been sitting here and listening to all the different codes being paged throughout the day. We had the fear that maybe something would happen here in the hospital. My mom said "If something happens, how do we get you out of here with all the machines?" She just kept pacing, trying to be on high alert. Our social worker came in to check on us, explaining we were safe and the hospital is trained in emergencies with patients like me. It didn't comfort us that much, but we had to believe.

As for the fundraiser, it's still in the process of being approved. Should be up next week at the latest and also, a good friend of mine has ordered bracelets, like the "LiveStrong" ones. These are in purple with my theme word, "Strength" and a heart. An L.M.M. heart, to help pay for expenses. When I finally get them in my possession, I will let you know. Day 45 and going strong.

Chapter 12
We Are Family

Wednesday, April 24, 2013

MOM, LAUREN AND DAD
FAMILY PHOT0

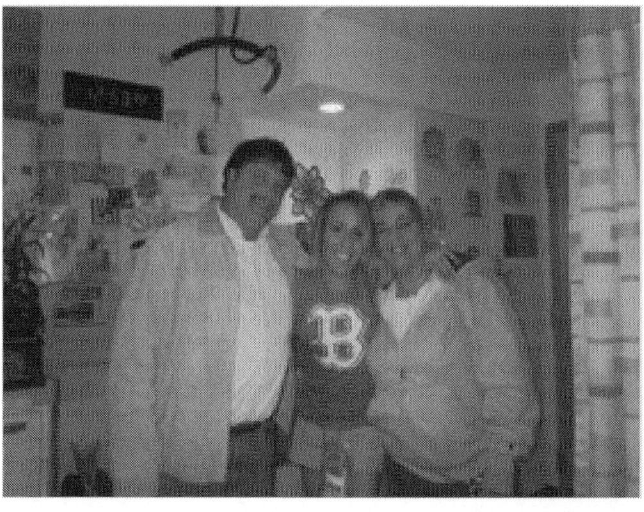

This picture was taken the last time Lauren was unleashed and my husband Dean was here. Today it is Day 10 and Lauren is having the PA line taken out. She will be mobile again. (God help the nurses.) They put her IV line in already, so we're just waiting for the doctor to come in and take the PA line out of her neck. SHOWER DAY!

When I look at this picture, I can't help but remember when Dean came into our lives. Lauren was only five years old. Today she is 22 but it seems like only yesterday when she was a little girl. We knew there were some medical problems, but nothing close to what it has turned-out to be.

I cannot thank my husband enough for all he has done for me and mostly our children. Being a blended family has its moments. Dean has a heart of gold and we, meaning Lauren and I, are so blessed to have him. I am the emotional one and Dean is the calm one, so together we have balance. We only get to see him on the weekends; he's at home during the week working and taking care of our dog, Ralfy. Every Friday he hops in the car straight from work to spend the weekend with us.

Together as a family, we are going to get
through this.
Sweetheart, we love you

Strength in Numbers
Thursday, April 25, 2013

Hello everyone,

Today is Day 51. Never thought we would be here this long. I sit and just stare out the window wishing a helicopter (the helicopter pad is right outside our window, I can see them coming and going) would land on the hospital pad with a heart for Lauren. As I look out the window, I watch people walking around, talking, laughing, moving on with their lives. I want that. All I can do is watch the world go by and pray my daughter stays stable. Inside, I am crying like hell, but not for anyone to see. Be Strong.

Today Lauren was supposed to have her PA line put back in but the nurse came in and told us "because she had had the line taken out so late yesterday and the cathe lab is backed up, they are going to say today is her full day off." Lauren was relieved; she isn't feeling that well. Upset tummy. I'm sure when she gets something to eat and then showers she will feel better. It is so hard to just sit here and watch her when she is not feeling well. The feeling of helplessness is so overwhelming. There are times when I will just get up and start dancing just to try to make her laugh. She says, "Mom, your losing it." To be honest, I have lost it.

Now on to another subject.... I ordered the wristbands. One of Lauren's friends designed them and they will be available around the first week of May. A lot of Lauren's friends said they wanted to create a wristband for Lauren so show support for her. The proceeds from the bands will go toward Lauren's financial obligations. We are blessed that she had good insurance but not for everything.

When Lauren receives her new heart, she will be starting a new life. I want to make sure that she is not financially strapped. She has been through so much, way too much.

Numerous people have been requesting the wristbands for themselves and to sell for Lauren. If you would like one or would like to sell some, please let us know. They are $5.00 each. Thank you for your support.

Lynne

Blanket of Love

Tuesday, April 30, 2013

Hello all,

This is the blanket that I'm making for Lauren from all the yarn that has been given to us. I cannot thank everyone enough; I haven't crocheted since I was in high school. Each color and row has a special message for Lauren. Even when I am working on it, I think about that person who gave us the yarn and why they selected it. Lauren has been directing me on which color goes next. So a big "THANK YOU," it really means a lot to us and helps to keep me busy. I'm so glad I decided to create this blanket, it's great therapy for me. Busy mind and busy hands.

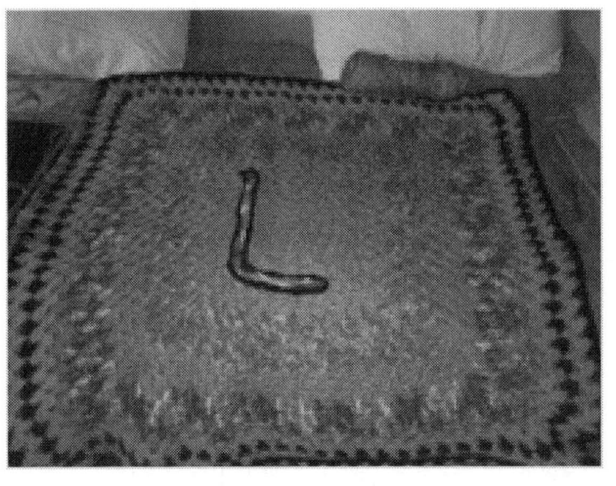

This is Day 56 and going strong. One day at a time.

I was so surprised to find out how many have been reading and following our online journal. I feel bad that we do not update more often. We will work on that. Please leave a comment, we love hearing the feedback.

So many times I feel alone, but I need to remember that I may be physically alone but not emotionally alone. I take comfort in knowing how many people love us, care for us, and are praying we come home soon.

Big thanks go out to all those friends that they told me they were worried about Dean. I will make sure he takes you up on all the dinner invites.

Love,
Lynne

Living Without Privacy

Tuesday, April30, 2013

This is a quick post that we needed to write. The hospital has posted a sign on our door "DO NOT ENTER, MUST SEE NURSE FIRST." The reason for the sign is that Lauren and I live here now. It's for our privacy and security. There are many times when people come up and just walk right in and Lauren is on the porta-potty, (It's on the side of her bed as soon as you walk in the room.) Or, at times she has been tired and not up for company; the same goes for me. I include myself in this issue; I do live here with her (she won't let me leave, I wouldn't either). This is our house, or home, whatever way you want to look at it. Lauren loves the company but there are times she is not up for it and we all know Lauren, she will not say anything until after the fact. So we ask everyone to respect the sign on the door and please check with the nurse before entering. There are also times when she is not properly dressed, if you get what I am talking about. So please do not just walk in, we wouldn't just walk into your house.

Love,
Lynne & Lauren

Lauren Speaks Up……
Wednesday, May 8 2013

The response with the selling of our bracelets has been mind-staggering. We initially ordered twelve hundred bracelets and we are most likely going to be needing to order more! I can't believe it. Thank you everyone, it brings tears to my eyes. People that don't even know me are showing their love and support. A boost I needed to keep strong.

Here's a little update from my point of view: we'll start with the good news. Mike (we went to school together) and I started dating and he is NOT scared about any of this. The nurses told me that stuff like this usually tears relationships apart because of all the emotional and financial issues that arise. I think I landed a good one.

Now, serious issues…The doctors told me in January that my heart was functioning at 30% and now judging by the numbers, it is at about 10%. In other words, I probably shouldn't even say this, but if I was to give up on this whole hospital deal, pack up, and go home, they say I would have a max of about two weeks to (ahem), live.

So with that said, looks like I am parking my butt at Brigham for a bit longer. The doctors have inserted a feeding tube through my nose and it sucks so bad. Put it this way, I don't even want my five-year-old niece to see me like this; I don't want to scare her. The feeling is like having a pill, or food, caught in the back of your throat. To make matters tougher, I'm on an extremely strict fluid restriction; in the course of a day, I can only have a total of 1.75L. That's less than a soda bottle of fluid, for the entire day. If it doesn't sound horrible, give it a try, especially all you eight-cups-of-coffee-drinkers.

With the feeding tube, it makes it worse; I'm constantly having dry mouth. I hate it. I have never been this upset in my life; and scared. OHHHHH and don't forget I still have a catheter in the left side of my neck and a catheter in my arm. No 22-year-old, hold on, let me rephrase that….no *person* should ever have to endure this much pain!

I still have no idea when I'll get a heart. I told my mom, "I wish I was dealing with this during September, then the weather would suck. It's May and my birthday is coming up, and the weather is nice."

I try to be optimistic. I never thought it'd be this soon or this hard. I feel like every day I'm losing more and more of my freedom. I know things could be worse. I mean, I was here during the bombing and could have been a part of that horrific event, but words can't even truly describe what it feels like. I know, "keep my eye on the prize," but most days the prize seems out of reach, not even obtainable. *Oh, shut up Lauren*, I know.

So to wrap it up cuz I'm tired, the doctors have deemed me EXTREMELY sick at this point and I'm considered more mal-nutritioned than a child in a Third World country. I have a feeding tube in my nose and I keep trying to pay my nurses off to remove it, LOL.

Love always & forever, Lauren

The Online Fundraiser Is Up
Friday, May 10, 2013

www.helphopelive.org

Type in Lauren Meizo under patients name and it will bring you to her page. This is a great web site that helps people with medical issues. Our social worker gave us all the information. A patient can only use the money for medical matters, so people feel that when they donate the money is used for the reason it's meant for.

Hmmmmmm….Life in The Hospital

Monday, May 13, 2013

Anyone who knows me well, knows that there are two things I love most in life, besides people and those are.. FOOD & LYING IN BED. I'm sick of both of them these days. I've learned what can happen to me when my body doesn't take in enough calories by mouth; an NG tube a/k/a, a feeding tube. My experience with that was nothing but hell! My brother Mikey told me I looked like Snuffleupagus, the elephant from Sesame Street. Yup, that's my brother for you. I was oddly and happily surprised that Madison, my niece, was not scared of me with all the wires and tubes coming out of me.

My brother and his family have made it a point to come up every other week, usually on a Friday after work. They come visit with me, then they take my mother out for dinner. With all my machines, my niece is not scared at all. She will just jump on my bed, ask questions, then say, "let's color."

Feeding tubes are not fun. They lubricate it up and ask you to keep sipping out of a cup of water fast, fast, fast, while it slides down into your stomach. Then they tape it to your nose. So basically, it's hard not to go crossed-eyed; you have this tube sticking straight out from your face the entire time.

During the day, it serves no purpose. It pumps twelve hours at night. You have to deal with the bullshit associated with it: constant headaches from the pressure, the feeling of a double ear infection, and a sore throat. You can actually see the tube when I open my mouth all the way. Maddie kept asking me to open my mouth to see it…what a weirdo.

Good news is, they finally took it out! Thank God. I had to make so many promises to eat, so they told me they will give it a try. I forced myself to eat to the pathetic point that I was out of breath. That's how bad things have gotten, how weak I am these days. I have extreme shortness of breath after sitting in freakin bed eating a yogurt. My mom has to push me to eat otherwise, now, I know she is losing it. She will stick a straw up her nose and say "do you want to look like this again?"

Life in a hospital: so when I came in here, there was snow on the ground and everyone was talking about how cold it was but now it's mid-May…almost my birthday, and as I look out the window, I just sigh. I tend to ask my mom to keep the blinds down as much as she'll allow. I'm not having a pity party, this is just my life at this point and for the most part, my mom's as well. I'll be blunt, I constantly tell my mom I wish this bullshit was happening in Sept/Oct., because the way I see it…I'll be spending summer healing.

I still have yet to read the transplant book in its entirely; I'm scared more than anything. I want to be able to swim and be in the sun (NO MORE BABY OIL, like I'm known for, LOL, I'm like a slip 'n slide during the summer). Spray-tan coupons as gift ideas for me…..wink, wink.

Each day, each hour, each minute, each second, I'm one step closer to my special gift of a new heart. My mother just sits here and prays and stares out the window talking with God, to keep her daughter safe. It could happen at any moment. I had a little scare the other day and thought maybe it was the day. I called for food and the woman on the other end told me I was in the computer as "NPO" -nothing by mouth. My mom went running to the nurse to find out what was going on. I was thinking, *am I soon headed in for open heart surgery?* False alarm. I guess I can look at it as a test of how I'll react when the time comes. I know my day will come eventually; until then I guess I just have to wait like I've been doing.

Sorry for not allowing any visitors for the past week or so. I really needed my rest. I'm getting weak. Hell, my mom gave me a sponge bath the other day and just washing up my heart rate hit 150 at times. My nurse joked afterward, once I was calmed down, and said "Jeez, are you running a marathon in here?"

My nurse Tom has to put up with me every shift he works; very smart man, knows his stuff but has no problem giving me shit back when I dish it out to him. He typically gets the long-term patients so he's stuck with my butt until I get my heart. He helps keep my spirits up, along with my mom.

Now her! That's a whole other story; I think the poor woman is losing her mind along with weight. It is very expensive to eat in a hospital so mom normally will eat only a bagel for breakfast, then a salad with tuna around 2pm. Then she says she is good for the day. She looks amazing these days, no lie. She and I are going to have to go clothes shopping after this ordeal. At this point, she'll do anything to put a smile (even if it's just a little smirk) on my face by dancing or singing, she's random! A big moment of the day for her is to take a walk in the morning. She will get a coffee then take a short walk outside around the hospital. She says it helps clear her mind for the day. She stays close to the hospital because there are a lot of crazies are out there. If it wasn't for her, I think I would have just given up. LOVE HER!

I would like to thank everyone for your support and prayers,
maybe tonight?

Love,
Lauren

I Want To Share a Beautiful Message
Thursday, May 16, 2013

Hello,This is Lynne; my husband sent me a beautiful message today. Lauren had her PA line put in this morning. I made a comment to my husband

"I'm tired of being alone" and this is what he said:

"What you're doing is amazing. She needs that support and you're always there for her. With that said, I understand the frustration. Just remember that I love you and will always be with you, even when I am not physically there. Love my two girls."

It just made me feel special and loved, giving me the encouragement to keep going strong.
Love you, sweetheart…

What's up, Lauren ?
Wednesday, May 22, 2013

So a storm is coming in today (weather-wise) and I decided to write to keep my mind busy. Great idea, Mom, it helps to get things out. A local hometown newspaper did an article about me. It was a phone interview. My mom contacted them. 'Local Woman in Need of a Heart Transplant, Living in a Hospital in Boston." She knows how to make me feel special, boosting my spirits.

When the article came out, I was front page. Right on the front was a large picture of me. I couldn't believe it. I'll sign your copy, it'll be worth $$$ one day, watch, you'll see, LOL.

> The bracelets have been spreading like wildfire! I'm truly amazed by how many people are willing to buy, wear, and sell them to help. They are in about six or seven states all down the East Coast. Organizing the bracelets from my hospital bed has been keeping my mind busy. My nurses laugh and say I am running a business; they have never seen something like this before. But they are all wearing one. When we get a request, I pack them up and my mom found a post office down the street, so she takes a walk and mails them out.

So what's been up with me? Today they mentioned that I may have to switch rooms to another one on this floor. HA! WHAT? Are they crazy? My decor is coming off the walls when it's time for me to take a trip on down to the 6th floor (pre-operation). The reason for this joke of an idea was, this past weekend, I had a short in one of the wires on my TV. Well, the TV and the rest of my monitors are all hooked up to pretty much in the same place. The nurses were unable to print the hourly strips they need for my PA line. Luckily they were able to fix it! There was no way I was leaving my beautiful room.

This afternoon, a lovely, elderly woman who goes around to say prayers with patients was attracted to my room by my colorful door with the pink flamingos on it. She came in and was completely mesmerized by my room and how it felt more homey and welcoming than a regular hospital room. She was so cute and kept asking me if I was a teacher, because she had been a kindergarten teacher and my room reminded her of all the decorations. While she was here, she gave Mom and I communion, which was very nice.

My mom noticed my IV (they had to put me back on IV Lasix, I had started retaining fluids again; I peed out 3 lbs since yesterday) was red and started to bleed. We wrapped my arm in a face cloth while waiting for the IV nurse to come. Well, a face cloth ended up not being enough…the lure lock that connects the IV tubing to the arm catheter came unscrewed and my arm started gushing blood. Mom was asked to step out of the room because of all the blood; she couldn't stop shaking and crying. The bleeding had to be controlled with a full-sized towel while the nurses took care of me. It didn't hurt a bit, just a huge mess. I am just grateful this did not happen when I was sleeping. Thank God Mom was there to notice it.

On that note, I need to share this….. my mother watches my monitors like she is watching a TV show. She calls it "the Medical Show." The nurses have even told her she will go crazy just staring at the monitors, but being stubborn, she continues to do it. Mom knows what all the monitors do and what the right readings should be, so if she sees something different she will inform the nurses. A couple of times I was in trouble and Mom caught it right away. They keep saying they will have to put her on the payroll.

Mentally and emotionally, I'm doing all right. Hanging in there, being me. There are a couple of personal matters that are bothering

me that I won't go into detail on, but I won't let them rain on my parade.

My birthday is Friday and I've been dreading it because I'm, well….here. I'll have my catheter in my neck….so I will be leashed. I won't be able to get up. I was hoping to have my cake in the family room, not happening. On top of it, my tenth day is Saturday, but because they don't do PA lines on the weekend, I'd need to wait until Sunday, but it's a holiday weekend, so I'll need to wait to have my day off on Monday. I could if I wanted to, have them take it out Saturday, but that would means I'd be going three days without it in, I'd be bumped down to a 1B stat., which can ultimately be the difference between me getting an available heart that comes up over someone else. So as long as there is no fever and the site looks great, we're keeping it in.

With summer approaching, I am getting a little upset. The weather is going to be nice and everyone will be enjoying the warm weather. Swimming, going to the beach, and so on.

That's all I have
Lynne

Happy 23rd Birthday, Lauren
Friday, May 26, 2013

May 24, 2013

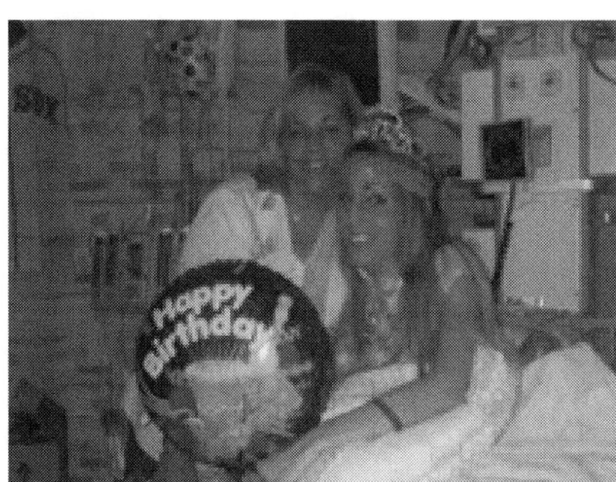

What a weekend. Our daughter turned 23 and if all of you know Lauren, she did it in style. We had a family gathering with Dean and myself, her brother Mikey, Katie and Maddie.

The day first started out with the whole transplant team of doctors coming into Lauren's room singing "Happy Birthday." Then, a little later, the nurses came in to sing "Happy Birthday" with a cake. Lauren had a surprise visitor: her friend Shannon (little sis) came with her friend Tiffany, with a cake. I have never heard that song sang so much in one day.

Okay, now a big surprise: Lauren received a special birthday wish from Remdog and Don from the Boston Red Sox. They sent her a video message wishing her a happy birthday and sending good thoughts that she will receive her new heart soon. Her smile was unbelievable (mine too). I didn't think I could make it happen but I met someone in the hospital that had a friend who worked for the Boston Red Sox. Didn't say a word to Lauren, just in case it didn't happen. When we received the video, Lauren was so surprised, I thought I was going to faint. Love those two guys. They took the time to wish my daughter a happy birthday.

Thanks to all for all the birthday wishes.

Wednesday, May 29, 2013

Today when I was taking my morning walk I came across a kind woman. She looked at me and said "you looked troubled." So I started telling her about my daughter and she stopped right there and said a prayer for Lauren, myself and our family. This woman, I found out, is a Boston policewoman, and took the time to talk with me. We sat for about an hour and chatted. I felt better; there are kind people in our world.

After I returned from my walk, it turned rainy and gloomy here today inside and out. I have a meeting with our transplant social worker and she is going to help me figure out all this insurance stuff. Apparently there has been some confusion in her insurance policy. Needed to call the company to confirm Lauren's insurance is all up to date. I have so many forms I need to fill out to make sure that Lauren will have the coverage she needs.

Always remember your social worker is your best friend if you are living in a hospital. They have all the resources you may need. Love ours……

Lynne

Faith, Believe, Hope
Thursday, May 30, 2013

These three words mean so much to me. My sister Donna put them over my couch bed. When I am lying down, I keep reading them and they give me the strength to make it another day.

A friend of ours from back home wrote a beautiful poem for Lauren. After we read it, we both cried; feeling the love in his words was overwhelming. It is so beautiful we would like to share it with everyone:

STRENGTH

Strength. I used to think strength was from lifting weights, toning your muscles to make you look great. I used to think strength was from working out. To shed off those inches all about, I now see the real 'strength' is in the mind. Fighting through life while being so kind, I truly believe that you will pull through. This world truly needs more people like you. For now I know this to be true, it is mental toughness, in my view. For the strongest person that I know, is the one we all love Lauren

By Russ Peltier

Day 84 and counting……

Friday, May 31, 2013

Today Lauren is not feeling well. Sleeping mostly and not really eating. I wish I could do something for her, except sit here and watch her heart monitor like it were a TV. I watch it all the time. Her heart is working so hard at this point, I get nervous. Lauren is so thin, you can see her heart beating against her skin, and so fast.

Went outside for a bit today and got depressed. So beautiful outside, Lauren and I should be home by the pool. Soon, we hope. Loneliness and despair are starting to hit me more and more. I would say depression, but I am so past that.

Tonight, if you look at the stars, say a prayer for Lauren, maybe if we flood the Lord with prayers he'll answer them

With much love,
Lynne

We need to smile again!
Day 93

Friday, June 7, 2013

Here we are on Day 93…..

I know this isn't a good picture, but we are still trying to smile. The only way I can express how we feel right now is we are playing bingo for the cover all and we are just waiting for one number before we can yell "BINGO!" Anxious, happy, nervous, just waiting. Well, that's how we feel. We are just waiting for our number to come. We want to yell BINGO, when they come into our room and say her heart is here.

Lauren hasn't posted too much, she is getting weaker and very tired. I can see it in her eyes, she's scared. I cannot take seeing my daughter slipping away from me. All I can do is sit with her, hold her hand and tell her "I'm sending you strength." *Lord, please help my daughter, I can't lose her.*

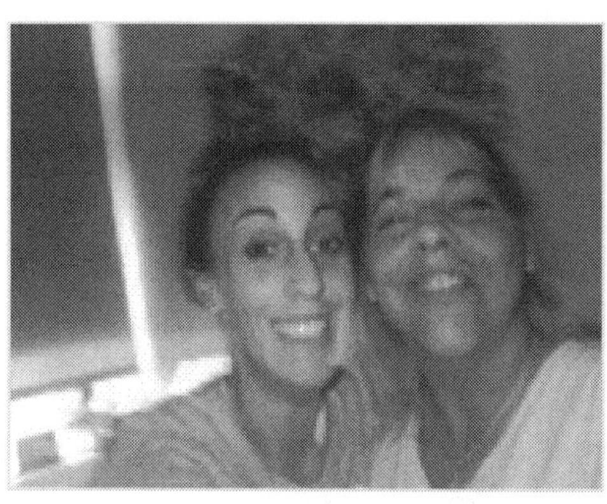

This photo was taken a week ago, when Lauren was unleashed. She always tries to put a smile on her face. But when you really look at it, I see

fear in her eyes. She has lost so much weight, I'm afraid they are going to put a feeding tube in her soon.

So many people die waiting on the transplant list; national figures say 22 people a day. My gut it telling me we are running out of time. *Please Dear Lord, give my daughter her second chance at life.* I find myself going to the hospital chapel more frequently. I cannot have Lauren see me losing it.

Please pray for my child.

Love,
Lynne

Chapter 13
Moved to ICU

Friday June 21, 2013

On June 13th Lauren was getting very sick, her heart was only functioning on her right side and the left side was deteriorating. News you don't want to hear, "We need to move Lauren to ICU today." I called my husband, explained what was happening and he told me "I'm on my way."

Lauren was very scared and in a lot of pain. Being in the ICU is a very frightening place to be. We had to pack Lauren's room up.. OMG, so much to pack. You can say we had a lot of stuff.

Walking into her new room we had to wear the yellow hospital gowns over our clothes. Each time you entered you had to put a new one on. The room was very sterile; it looked like a hospital room on steroids. Lauren's nurse had a station right in the room. She was in there with us at all times. I told Lauren I was not leaving her, so they allowed me to sleep in her room. No way was I leaving her alone. My husband had to sleep in the family room; we were told only one family member was allowed to spend the night in ICU.

Watching Lauren being hooked up to all the machines, the nurses would glance at my husband and I with concerned expressions on their faces. I knew it was not good. We sat quietly, holding hands, feeling totally helpless. My thoughts kept going, *we are all leaving this hospital together. No way did we sit in this hospital all these months to end up like this. Lauren will get better.* I had to believe; without hope I would have nothing.

We were approached by the doctors on Saturday June 15th. Lauren needed to have surgery; they were going to have to surgically insert a balloon in her heart to keep it pumping. We were told they would perform the surgery the following morning, Father's Day. I was handed the consent forms to sign because at this point, I had to become Lauren's Health Care Proxy. Lauren was in no condition to make decisions anymore. I stood there looking at the paper, shaking. I was told that after they performed the surgery they were going to keep her sedated, a medically-induced coma. When they insert the balloon she cannot move and the only way to achieve that would be to keep her heavily sedated. My poor baby was getting so sick her organs were starting to be affected. After listening to all the doctors, and a lot of crying and praying, there was no other choice.

I knew that Sunday morning would be the last time I would be able to talk with Lauren for a while. That evening was so hard, praying the surgery go well, wondering how long my daughter would have to stay sedated. She was heavily medicated to help with her pain. A couple of times she would slightly open her eyes and I would say, "I'm here," then she would go back to sleep. I kept thinking, *will I ever talk to Lauren again? See her walk? Oh hell, live? I'm sitting here watching my daughter die right in front of me. Lord help us, please..*

Morning of Lauren's surgery: last time I will be able to talk with her for who-knows-how-long. I told Lauren I will be by her side at all times. I told my daughter that while she is sedated I will make sure that she is treated with dignity and respect at all times. That was my promise to her. She looked at me and Dean with tears in her eyes and I whispered in her ear "stay strong, you're my little Pollock and we do not give up." With a slight smile on her face, they wheeled her out of the room. At that point, I just fell into my husband's arms and cried uncontrollably.

After what seemed like forever, after three hours, we received the news we wanted to hear. Lauren was out of surgery and doing fine. All I kept thinking, and I know Dean was as well, was *she's alive. We still have our daughter.* When we were finally able to go see her, our hearts just weren't ready for what we saw. Lauren had two machines keeping her alive.

This surgery was only a temporary fix; Lauren would not be able to stay in this state for a lengthy period of time, waiting for a new heart. She would need to have a LVAD implanted in her heart called, HeartWare. They call this the new bridge to transplant.

The HeartWare System will help Lauren's weakened heart pump blood throughout her body. The pump, called an HVAD pump, circulates blood by moving it from the left side of her heart and pumping it into her aorta (the large blood vessel that carries blood from her heart to the rest of her body). The pump is inserted into the heart and two small motors inside the pump circulate the blood. A driveline exits her skin next to her belly button and connects the pump to a controller. The controller operates the pump and tells us if there are any problems with the system. It all runs on batteries. Lauren will need to carry a battery pack with her at all times.

With no time to waste, they scheduled the surgery for June 18th; the following Tuesday.

Chapter 14

Bridge to Transplantation Begins

June 17, 2013

The night before the surgery, all of Lauren's doctors came by and when they started to give me hugs, I was really scared. It felt more like they were stopping in to say goodbye.

I was sitting in the hallway looking out a window, just staring into the night numbly when one of Lauren's doctor came and just sat with me. I looked at her and s, "Lauren is going to be okay, right?" Her answer: "Lauren is very sick, she needs to make it through aid the night." She hugged me for quite a while. At that moment, I realized I could really lose my daughter. *Oh my God, Lauren is dying*. In my mind, yes, I'd had thoughts about that but never wanted to believe the truth. That hug gave me the truth. That evening Dean and I sat next to Lauren all night, talking to her. Even though she was sedated, I knew in my heart that she could hear us.

June 18th is here.

The surgery that Lauren was having was not at Brigham & Women's Hospital. She had to be moved to a different hospital due to her small frame size. The VADs at Brigham & Women's were too large for her small frame. Meeting with the surgeon, he explained to us that patients do move to different hospitals in order to match their needs. Most of the hospitals are in the same area and many have underground halls connecting them. They would be able to move her with all her machines right into the operating room of a different hospital.

Lauren had the first surgery. They surgically inserted a balloon in her heart to keep it pumping. That was just a temporary fix to keep her alive, then the next surgery was to insert the LVAD called HeartWare, and have the balloon taken out.

The HeartWare System helps Lauren's weakened heart pump blood throughout her body. The pump, called the HVAD pump, circulates blood by removing it from the left side of her heart and pumping it into her aorta (the large blood vessel that carries blood from her heart to the rest of her body). The pump is inserted into the heart and two small motors inside the pump circulate the blood. A driveline exits her skin and connects the pump to the controller. The controller operates the pump and tells us if there are any problems with the system. Lauren will need to carry a battery pack with her at all times.

As the clock ticked before they took her, I thought, *Lauren is going to undergo surgery again. The bigger surgery, open heart surgery.* We were told that people could stay on the balloon pump and wait for a heart, but in Lauren's case, she needed this procedure done. Again I was handed the consent forms to sign. Being Lauren's health proxy I have to make decisions and sign consent forms for her when she is unable. Even though she is my child and an adult, I am her legal guardian at this point. When she becomes conscious she will be able to make decisions on her own. Dean and I were faced with the most important decision a parent can make. Lauren will be only the third person to have this device inserted to date. The other patients are doing well and one has received a new heart.

At this point we really didn't have a hard decision to make: without this new surgery she didn't have a chance. She would die.

We signed.

Right before they took her through the doors to the surgical unit, I stopped them and again whispered in her ear "stay strong, you're my little Pollock and we do not give up." When they wheeled her in and the doors closed, I just broke down crying and praying that God would keep her safe. She is too young, too beautiful, and too strong with a will to live a happy life. My husband and I just held each other. No words.

Our two wonderful friends, Russ and Cheryl surprised us, taking the day off from work to be with us. It really meant so much to us and they helped us pass the time. Talking and crying, Russ has a way of making us laugh. Love you guys so much.

When Lauren was in surgery, I kept praying that she stay alive. Open heart surgery was very risky for her, going in as sick as she is. We were told the surgery was going to take around six hours. It was very comforting to have our friends with us.

As we were sitting in the waiting room, the surgeon came out. My first thought was, *you are here too early, oh my God, no.* I just looked at him and asked, "Is Lauren alive?" He told us that she was alive and had done very well. This doctor and his team gave Lauren her life back. He also told us he took a sample of tissue from her heart that did not look normal, for testing.

When Lauren was brought up to her room in the ICU and all situated, we were finally able to see her. I was not prepared. Tubes and monitors, machines beeping, so many machines, all attached to her. She was still on a breathing machine and I was so afraid of tripping on something. They told me I could stay with her, so my new bed was a cushion on a window sill. That was fine, I wasn't expecting to sleep much anyway.

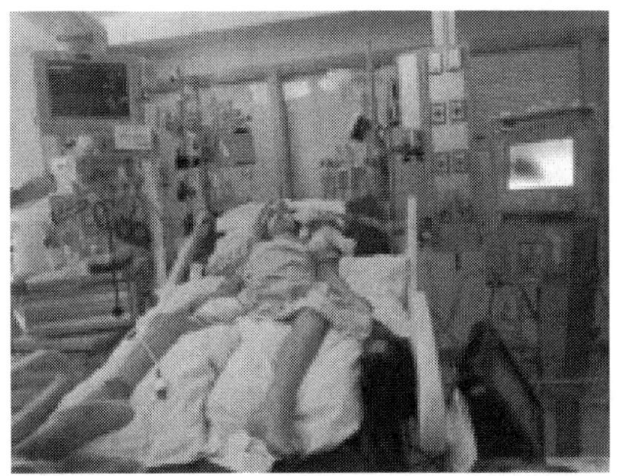

The next day, the surgeon approached us and told us the test had come back on the tissue sample; one of Lauren's ICD lines had become infected and her defibrillator would need to come out. That would bring us to surgery number three.

After just having had open heart surgery, now they had to go back in and remove the infected ICD. A couple of days later, they had to get her stable enough for the operation. We had quite a few scares after the second surgery; they couldn't get her stabilized. You know something is wrong when the red lights on the monitors go off and all the doctors and nurses rush in. I just remember Dean holding me in his arms and the both of us crying, when they yelled "get the crash cart!" It's a position I would never wish on anybody. Lauren had two more episodes like that. Heavily sedated, in a coma, she had no idea what was happening. I would talk to her and hold her hand to give her the STRENGTH she needed to get through this.

Lauren has undergone three surgeries in one week, all very scary. I whispered in her ear, "they do not make enough moisturizer to take away the worry wrinkles." Every time she went into surgery, I reminded her, "you are my strong Polish girl, be strong."

I have not talked with Lauren in two weeks. She has been sedated the whole time. She had woken up a few times (they would lift the sedation just slightly, periodically) and would look at us but she shouldn't talk with the breathing tube in. We are hoping it will come out soon. We are not out of the woods yet. Before, we were living our lives one day at a time, but these days it is one hour, one minute, at a time.

The LVAD is working great in Lauren's heart.

Big Relief.

Tuesday July 2, 2013

It has been three weeks since I've written about Lauren's condition. Sorry. So after three weeks in the ICU, they've started to lift some of the sedation. To me, it was like Christmas morning to be able to look into Lauren's eyes and say "hello there."

She can't talk; she still has the breathing tube in. We found ways to communicate and are getting very good at cha-
rades.

Lauren has been experiencing what they call "ICU successes." With all the meds she's on, she's been hallucinating some of the time. But we got through that. My job right now is to make sure she is safe, cared for, and comfortable, but most of all to give her encouragement that we are going home soon. When I tell her that, she smiles.

Everything that has happened to Lauren is not right, not fair. Every night I lay here in the hospital with her and pray that tomorrow is a better day. It seems things are changing all the time. Our big fight now is to strengthen her lungs so the breathing tube can come out. The doctors told me they are going to try on Friday. So please, pray that her lungs will be strong enough.

I am so done with living in the hospital. If I go outside, I'm tired of walking down the hall, I feel like everyone is watching me. When I reach the elevator I pray no one is in there, just to have a few moments alone. When I sleep, I can't just close the door; nurses are always in the room, no privacy at all. Lauren and I missed spring time and it looks like we will probably miss summer. You know, yes, it bothers me, but I will do whatever it takes to get my daughter better no matter how long it takes. Until then we will have to be STRONG POLISH WOMEN LIKE MY MOTHER TAUGHT ME TO BE AND I WILL DO IT

TOGETHER WITH
LAUREN.

Lynne

Chapter 15

What the Hell is on the Back of Lauren's Head?

July 3, 2013

Lauren has been living in the ICU in a medically-induced coma and on life support. Sitting there day in and day out just looking at her, praying and talking to her was the norm. Nursing staff coming and going. My accommodations consisted of a mat on the window sill next to her bed. As a mother, you do what you need to do.

I was helping the nurse clean Lauren up when I noticed the back of her head. I screamed, "What the hell is that on the back of Lauren's head?" There was this huge, deep black mass on the back of her head; no hair, just a large bald spot with this large black spot; I really am finding it hard to describe. Let's just say it looked like a black scab.

The nurse looked at me with fear in her eyes and said "I will be right back." Thank God Lauren was sedated or I'd have scared her.

The nurse came back into the room and told me that Lauren had developed a pressure sore. I looked at her and said "What?? How did this happen?" She explained it, saying it developed from her head not being repositioned, turned or rotated. I then checked her whole body. I did find another one that was on her lip. Never noticed it before, but now I knew what I was looking for. I looked at her lip where the ventilator hose was from the breathing machine and found a small

black spot. They never slid it from side to side. I never touched it (didn't know it just slides from side to side).

I could not stop shaking at how gross it looked. There's my baby laying there, and now this. Unacceptable. I was so happy I found the two sores but now what do we do? Plus, all the hair loss. Lauren is going to freak out. I feel so bad, I let her down. I keep thinking of the promise I made to her, *I will keep you safe.*

A few nurses came in to the room to look at Lauren's head and told me this happens. I said "Not to my daughter. Why? Just tell me why." I wished I'd known about this; I would have moved her head and vent hose myself.

They proceeded to put some ointment and a badge on her head. They couldn't get the bandage to stick, so they would just position her head on it. They called the plastic surgery department to come evaluate it. When they showed up, they said they would put a plan of action to together for the sore.
A couple of days went by and nothing. I kept asking the doctors and the nurses what the plan would be. All I kept getting was "I'll look into it."

At this point, I felt I needed to call Lauren's transplant team to inform them of what was going on. Our nurse practitioner came to see us. She told me that she will contact the transplant team to keep

them posted and she would call plastic surgery at Brigham's about the pressure sore. I felt better with them in the loop.

When Lauren had her first surgery on June 18th, she was taken off the transplant list. So to this day, she is still off the list because of the LVAD surgery. She will not be placed back on until she is healthy enough.

I received a call from Brigham's saying that Lauren's transplant doctor is very concerned about her sore. It might take a while for it to heal and she cannot undergo her heart transplant with any open wounds at all due to possible infection. I felt like I was kicked in the stomach; all that waiting and now with everything I have to worry about, let's just throw her another wrench. Stay focused, let's get her off the breathing machine.

I need to talk with her, I feel so alone.

Friday July 5, 2013

They tried to take the breathing tube out today but being sedated for so long, Lauren lost almost all muscle tone, which includes her lung function. This leads us to surgery number four.
Lynne

Monday July 8, 2013

Lauren had to have a tracheotomy. A tracheotomy is an opening surgically created through the neck into the trachea to allow direct access to the breathing tube. A tube is placed through this opening to provide an airway, connected to an oxygen machine. At this point, she will not have anything in her mouth, so we will be able to talk again. Once again, more consent forms.

All went well but I hated to see the collar around her neck with a tube sticking out. My Lord, how many things does she have to endure?

Lynne

Just Love This Picture
July 16, 2013

When I look at this picture, I have so many different feelings. Love would be at the very top; it makes me smile and I

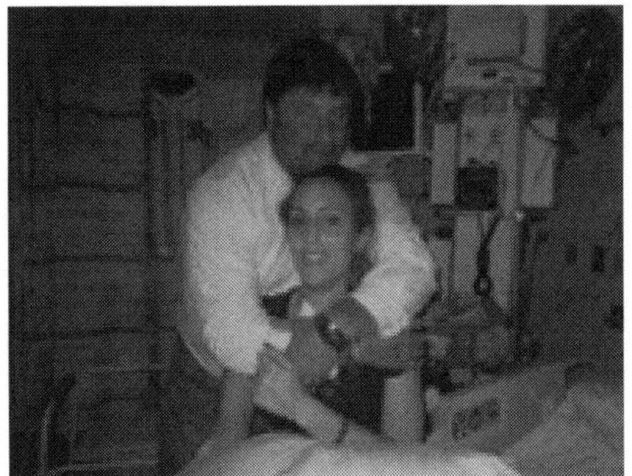

want Lauren to look this happy again.
Right now she is making great strides to get herself stronger. We have a long way to go but every little baby step is what we live for. Today she sat on the edge of the bed (with help), but it's her first time sitting straight up. We were so excited. Today she did her physical therapy three times and they only wanted her to do it once. That's my little Pollock…..she is not giving up.

My heart aches for her every minute of every day but we smile and sometimes we cry together. We pinky-swear to each other we are going home.

Love always,
Lynne & Lauren

Saturday July 27, 2013

Lauren is getting stronger every day. Yesterday she had the feeding tube removed from her nose and now has it in her stomach; she needs the extra calories. So she has no tubes or anything on her beautiful face now.

Today is a beauty day: eyebrows and make-up. Good therapy for her. Working with her hand coordination. Good reason to start doing something to make her feel better about herself.

I told her she's going to write the next post; she has to start communicating with all her friends so I said "you write one."
Love Lynne

Chapter 16

Out of ICU

158 days
Saturday, August 10, 2013

I know that on my last post I said that Lauren was going to write the next one. Well, I never know how Lauren is going to feel. Today is not a good day, she told me to write it for her. But I promise she will write a post soon, it's important for her to get some of her feelings out.

When we were transferred out of ICU, we both felt like there was a light at the end. It has been a long, hard journey. Lauren has been doing great; eating and even learning how to walk again. My daughter is back.

Yesterday they capped her trache; they had to see if she can go 24 hours breathing on her own and she's done it. So the plan is to have the trache removed; we need to go back to ICU to have this done and she needs to stay there 24 hours to be closely monitored. It's Christmas again.

During the past couple of months, Lauren has had to endure everything we were told "could happen."

As far as her pressure sore, she is being treated by a doctor at Brigham's Hospital. She had to endure treatments of him debrieding it to heal. We would put her in a wheelchair and wheel her from hospital to hospital for her visits. We are still waiting for the news that she is back on the transplant list. After all this time we still haven't received what we came here for: a heart.

During our time here, we've had a chance to reflect on a lot of things. Lauren's eyes were really opened as to what people are made of; good and bad. And there have been some bad. They know who they are, and we've decided to put that behind us and move forward, concentrating on all the people who have been there. We cannot say thank you enough for all the fundraisers, benefits, bracelet sales, and most of all, keeping us in your thoughts and prayers. Through this, Lauren and I have a closer relationship than we probably would've had before.

Love,
Lynne & Lauren

Lauren is Finally Outside Today!

Tuesday, August 13, 2013

Today Lauren was finally able to walk on the grass. The hospital has a small garden. This was her first time outside in two and a half months. Big Day. Of course, we had a doctor with us.

Lauren was standing in front of a wishing fountain and we didn't have a penny on us. I said, "do you want me to take one out of the fountain so you can make a wish?" She said, "Mom, really?" Anything for a laugh.

We sat outside on a bench for a bit before she got overwhelmed and started to cry thinking of all the seasons she's missed. We sat and talked and she felt better but was tired, so it was time to go back in. Also, the trache is out!

Tomorrow Lauren and I and her doctor are going out of the hospital. We need to start our training with the LVAD. First step is being outside the hospital supervised by our doctor. So Lauren said shopping. We decided to go to Marshall's. She was so excited to leave the hospital plus her favorite thing in the world… SHOPPING!!

The HVAF saved her life, now we still need to get the new heart so she can go on with her life…
Love, Lynne

Hi, It's Lauren

Wednesday, August 21, 2013

Yes, this is Lauren typing again but to be honest, I don't know what to write about. I missed out on so much of my life; as my mother explained, I had surgery after surgery, then spent over a month in a coma. I lost out on spring, summer, our family beach trip, and life's adventures.

Anyway, so yeah, I was completely out of it. Now I have a feeding tube in my stomach, an LVAD attached to me in the hip with a slit down my chest from surgery, and I have to carry this semi-heavy bag that has two batteries and a monitor (keeping the left side of my heart pumping, keeping me alive). I have three bullet-sized scars from where the blood needed to drain from the LVAD, life-saving surgery. That's right: *life saving,* without it I would have died because the left side of my heart was failing. I had to have Mom, nurses, and doctors try to explain what I went through, how sick I actually was.

I want to take a second to personally thank my mother for always being by my side and basically giving up her own life to stay by my bedside no matter what contraption she had to sleep on. She stuck up for me when the time was needed, signed consent forms when I was sedated, and held my hand every time they did blood draws, removed tape from my skin, and especially when I cried. I love you, Mom. You're my rock. You're my strong Pollock. Love Lauren

Lauren
Thursday, August 22, 2013

I came across this picture of Lauren; it was taken just before she got

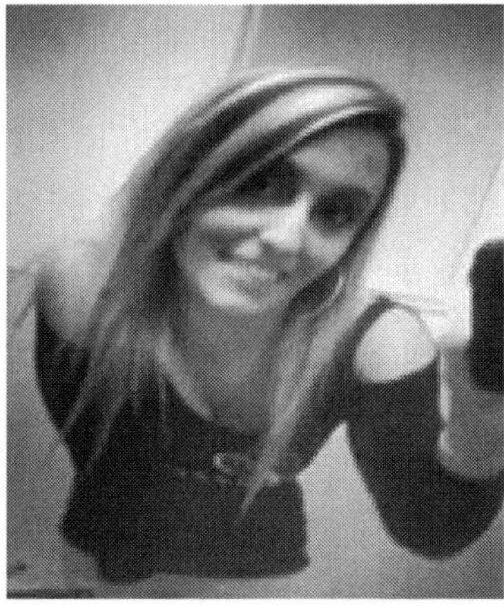

sick. Tomorrow we are going home. She is just as beautiful now as she was then.

She may have a few more battle scars but those are scars of bravery, courage, and determination. Not many people have it in them to endure everything she has gone through in the past 170 days. She is alive and going strong.

We came to Boston on March 6 to get a heart. Now we are going home on August 23 without what we came for. Lauren is very upset and says, "all that time in the hospital and I didn't get what I needed."

I keep telling her she was very sick and yes, we did wait, but during our waiting she needed to have open heart surgery to have the LVAD inserted. I will be taking care of her, so we will still be together all the time. I need to be with her. I am trained to take care of the controller and batteries for the LVAD machine.

In the past month I have been put through so much training, I feel like I've gone to medical school. I will need to know every aspect of the VAD and also proper care of her trache hole. Plus administering medication, both oral and shots. I also needed to complete a course in CPR, how to take her blood pressure, and check her sugar levels. Every day I will need to log all of her numbers and send them to the hospital every day on the computer.

My husband contacted our electrician to place an outlet on its own breaker in Lauren's bedroom for her. She will need to plug her controller in every night.

Friday, August 23, 2013
WE ARE GOING HOME TODAY

NOTHING MORE TO SAY, WE ARE GOING HOME !

I guess we will wait for the heart at home. Still waiting for the news that Lauren is a 1A on the transplant list.

Dean called me and said "On my way to pick-up my girls and bring them home.

Chapter 17

HOME SWEET HOME, FINALLY

Thursday, September 19, 2013

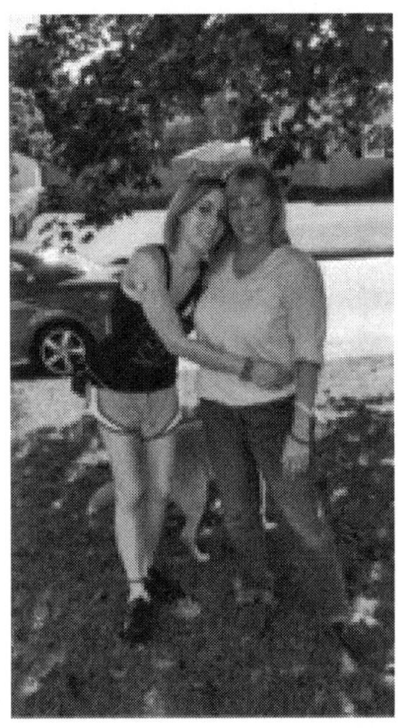

It's been a while, sorry.

Where to begin?

This is Week Four of being home. Time is passing so fast. I remember when Lauren and I were in the hospital, I would tell her that this is all going to be a memory someday. Just today we were looking at the blanket that I knitted for her with all the different yarns from everyone. She said "Mom, it seems like so long ago, me lying in the hospital bed watching you knit this blanket." I had to agree.

One thing I really need to say is there is nothing like sleeping in a bed. Every night is like sleeping on a cloud. I will never underappreciate the comfort of a bed again.

Our days have been very busy at home. We are blessed to have a wonderful team of nurses that come to the house to help me care for Lauren. Every day they come to help with her dressing changes. She has her VAD line in and we have to be extremely careful with this line since it goes directly into her heart. She still has a feeding tube because we need to keep her nutrition up, so every night I have to set up her feeds for her on the machine. Also, she has the wound on the back of her head. We went to the plastic surgeon last week and he was finally able to close it up. We go back to Boston on Friday; the surgeon wants to make sure it is healing properly. We go back next week to have the stitches taken out.

Every day I have to record Lauren's weight, temp, INR (from a blood test we do at home), and her numbers from the VAD controller, sending them all to her doctor in Boston; they are keeping a very close eye on her. We have a great team of doctors and nurses that I can call or text any time. We don't feel alone; we are in very close communication with the bonus of being at home.

It's great being home but we do travel to Boston once or twice a week. I don't mind; it gives me peace of mind when the doctors say Lauren looks great and all her numbers look good too. (So I guess I am doing something right.)

I am so proud of my daughter for everything she's had to go through and for everything still ahead. I am not sure if a lot of people would have the strength to endure the pain, frustration, and confusion in losing all her independence as she still waits for her heart.

When I mention independence, I don't just mean when she was in the hospital; now at home, Lauren cannot be left alone either. Dean, Lauren's boyfriend Mike, and myself, have all had to go through a training seminar on how to take care of her VAD controller. If Lauren was in trouble, (her heart) the controller has different alarms that would go off.

One of the biggest problems that Lauren has experienced is what they call "a suction event;" that is when the VAD will get suctioned to the wall of her heart and blood cannot flow. When that happens, (I freak, quietly to myself) Lauren needs to change her position and drink fluids. The first time it happened at home, I couldn't stop shaking after we got her out of it. But with time now, I'm a pro. I am CPR-trained now also; something I should have done a long time ago. I feel like I graduated from medical school, all the special training I had to have to be able to bring Lauren home.

There is so much more I would like to share, and I will. My thoughts at times go in so many directions, I want to make sure that I make sense when I write.

More to come…

Thursday, September 26, 2013

There's no place like home; it's not just a saying, it's truly a feeling.

Every day, we have a nurse come to the house to help with Lauren's care. She comes to do daily checks and helps with showering. I have been trained in all aspects of her care but the hospital set us up with visiting nurses. It's just a great comfort to have professional medical eyes here. We are so blessed to have three of the most caring, supportive nurses assigned to us. Most importantly, Lauren feels very comfortable with them.

We travel to Boston once a week at least, but this week we went on Monday to see the LVAD doctor and we go back on Friday to have the stitches taken out of her head from the pressure sore she had closed by a wonderful plastic surgeon. After that, we can only pray that her transplant surgeon will give us the thumbs up to do the heart transplant when a heart becomes available. I say that because he told us he would not do the surgery until it her head is healed and closed.

It has been great being back home but I know in the back of my mind that we will be back in the hospital when we get the call saying "we have a heart." There are times I watch Lauren going about her normal activities and I cry to myself remembering back to when she was in the hospital, hooked up to all the lines and listening to the beeps from all the monitors. The image of her in ICU is so clear in my mind. I know she needs her new heart and we'll have to travel that road again to be able to come home for good, but I'm not emotionally ready to relive those emotions yet. Then I wonder if Lauren feels the same. We have talked about it and we pray that it happens soon but we need to really find our strength to be able to go through it all over again.

Love,
Lynne & Lauren

Thursday, October 3, 2013
It's Lauren…It's October…One Year Since This All Began…

So I have been telling myself I need to get on and write a post for three reasons: 1) to give Mom a break for once, 2) to inform everyone of what is going on, on a more regular basis, and 3) to get my feelings out during this experience

Well, I lie in bed sometimes with a million ideas about what I want to talk about in my post and all my ideas just get mixed up so I apologize if I seem all over the place. My feelings are every which way; a lot of them I keep bottled up, so just work with me (LOL).

From a medical standpoint, the transplant team had their meeting, so Mom and I are just waiting for our phones to ring with the news as to where I stand on the transplant list - try to avoid prank calling us right now. We literally run to our phones when they ring.

For those of you who may be confused and thought I was already listed, well I am, but when I had my life-saving surgery, the VAD, I developed a pressure sore on the back of my head about 4 mm circular. The transplant surgeon did not want to do surgery on me if a heart became available because of two things: I'd be lying on the sore again during recovery (which could result in it growing larger and/or developing additional medical issues) and secondly, post-transplant I will be on steroid immune-suppressants, meaning my immune system will be greatly compromised and healing would take at least a year.

So, long story short, I have an amazing plastic surgeon who was able to close the wound by pulling the skin together- he will later fix my ugly trache scar! PHEW! So getting back to the "listing" bullshit: since I have an LVAD surgically implanted inside my heart, I'm currently a "1B" status. The phone call we are waiting for is to tell us I am a "1A," the top. Essentially, this means they believe I'll get a heart much faster. There is one rule though: I'd be a 1A for "30 free days." On the 31st day, they'd have a meeting again to discuss my standing, blah blah blah, everything is so technical!

How am I holding up? I'm doing about as well as you'd imagine. Some days are harder than others and I pull the "why me?!?" angry/jealous card, while others, I am in a great, bubbly mood. A few of my good friends redid my bedroom for me, something I have wanted to do since before hospital life. Thank you, guys!

Now it's just decorating; purple and black zebra w/silver, so fitting.

The boyfriend and I are doing great, I must say….like I've said before, most guys would've zipped out the door. Hell, I didn't know until like a month ago that while I was in a month-long coma, he came up, took a week off from work and just spent it with my boring ass..

Like I said though, this is hard work. I cannot be alone- meaning I always have to have someone close , just my family because they are trained on the device.

People typically wouldn't expect that I lack a pulse or wouldn't know that I can't ever have CPR performed on me because it could dislodge the device that's keeping the one side of my heart going. I am very blessed that I had the chance for this device. Fun fact: I'm the only one in western Mass. with this type; they're fairly new.

I have so much I want to talk about but don't know what to say. Ever since all of this hospital stuff began, especially after the surgeries and more invasive procedures, the scarring has really gotten to me. I hide how I feel most of the time, but I'm a 23 year old female with a slit down my chest, three "bullet holes" (hoses that were placed in my chest for drainage after the surgery), the ugliest frigging trache scar for everyone to see, and the PA line "hickey", with more that I won't even mention. I'm tired of people telling me "it's just a scar and it shows what you've been through and how brave you are." Yeah, you're right on that one…I'll give ya that, but have you ever thought this yourself or do you have a stupid scar to constantly remind you? You can look away and the scar is gone…I can't. It reminds me of when I had six full-grown adults move 107 lbs of me to a chair or when I had to learn how to walk and talk again. I'm still challenged by stairs every day and I've been out of surgery for months.

Not to mention my life. I don't know what was real or fake, my apologies, I guess I had some psychosis or something. Basically weird dreams, but with that, I'll only say in my head I thought my sweet nurse was going to kill me so I kicked her and had to be told of the event.

Wow, that felt good… even if it was just the tip of the iceberg. I won't express my feelings on certain topics, by the way. Sadness is all I can say.

Thank you, Love Lauren

Great News

Saturday, October 5, 2013

WE RECEIVED THE CALL

Lauren is now a "1A!"

Top of the heart transplant list again, we have been waiting since June. Lauren's transplant team has deemed her healthy enough to endure a heart transplant surgery.

Now we can get the call for a heart at any time...

Love,
Lynne

I'm sick of being sick......!
Sunday, October 13, 2013

When I was in the hospital, I was constantly told by every doctor, nurse, staff member and of course, friends and family - that I needed to talk and they'd listen. They did and I would like to say thank you, but I feel there are certain times I can complain about my aches and pains aloud, or better yet, to one person: my mom.

So this time, I've just decided to write to feel better, whether publicly or with a pen and my journal. So I type... I hope I do not offend anyone in any way; these are just some of my feelings - the feelings of a patient chronically ill with intense pain throughout her whole body, who in fact, is surviving this thing we call life with her heart controller hanging off her side like a pocketbook while waiting for a completely new one.

This isn't easy, I will say, and no one expects it to be, but it is far more intense than they discuss with you before discharge. I've been home now for a little over a month and the anxiety of how much longer I will have this machine in me. I am 23 year old now and I have to be treated like a child again. What I mean by that is, I can never be home alone so there is a lot of compromising with my mom. I cannot drive and actually, like a bad girl, I begged my mom to let me do it the other day and that stern Polish woman followed the rules and said no.

Let's see what else…oh yeah, I can't just hop in the shower or take a bath with the jets. I need the nurse to wrap me up, covering the drive line (wire to my heart), then hold the bag for me. And now that I'm a 1A and we're waiting for the call, I can't be more than 3 hours away from Boston for when the call comes. Basically, is anyone a good babysitter and looking for a job? Submit your resumes to my mom, because remember I can't be alone… sorry for the sarcasm, LOL.

Another thing that kind of annoys me when it comes to the medical staff with this transplant mumbo jumbo: they actually have no idea how the patient feels or what's going through our heads. They can tell us what to expect and what's to happen, they do lay out a great road map of the transplant process, I will definitely give them that, but none of them know what it's like. If I say I'm in pain, I'm in pain…I can't be told differently. That's like someone going through cancer; I can't tell them what emotions are right and which are wrong (also, at the same time, the thought of having a transplant is a foreign idea to most with little background knowledge, whereas cancer is sadly everywhere.)

I guess what I am trying to say is, if I don't feel well, I don't feel well, and that's pretty much the reason why I picked up my laptop to type. I'm sick of being sick! 2013 had to be, by far, the worst year, from a medical perspective. Hell, I met my Prince Charming through this and saw the true colors of those I thought were my closest friends and at the same time became closer with others.

When my mom and I said "Happy New Year 2013" to each other, we had no idea that only six short months later I'd be literally on my death bed undergoing emergency open heart surgery where she'd be asking the doctor if I was alive.

I hate to be a Negative Nancy; I'm just in one of those moods where I need to express that sometimes I'm not as strong as everyone thinks. I mean, I don't mean to toot my own horn, but with everything combined, and even just a day of chronic pain, I don't know many who could put up with all this and still smile, like this captain over here *TOOT* * TOOT*

I'm going to end this on a positive note. I want to thank everyone who came to my bowling event. They raised a good amount of money for my medical expenses. Thank you! Keep wearing those purple bands, guys. With your help I'll get through this without any complications.

Also as a side note, Mom and I want to spread the awareness about being a donor and how important it is to the person and family being blessed with the organ. Lots of families find peace knowing their loved one is going on to help someone else get better and continue to live out their life. All I'm saying is, consider getting that little red heart on the bottom of your license whether you think it's cute to have it there and believe in donors or you believe in this amazing and beautiful process.

In my case, when I do receive the heart I have to wait one full year until I'm able to contact the family of the donor. It is their choice whether they wish to contact me back or would rather not. Some people want to know who their organ came from and on the flip side, some families would like to know who is enjoying the precious gift. While in the hospital I was told some beautiful stories of the two parties meeting. For example, the donor's family came to the recipient's wedding! But since the system is so confidential, in some cases, no one wants to know anything. I have already decided I'd like to contact my donor's family & thank whoever they are.

Lots of Love Lauren

Family Time
Friday, October 18, 2013

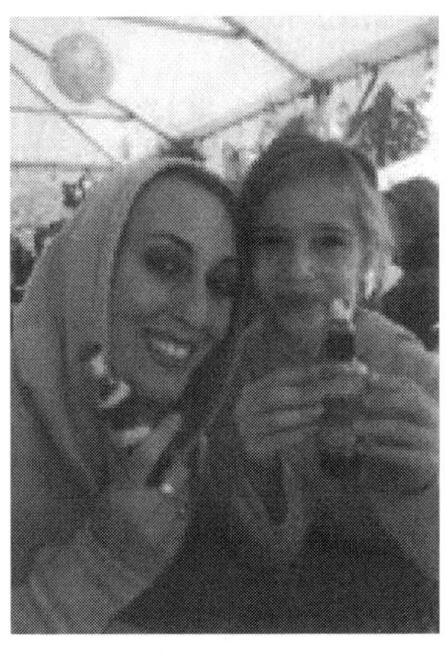

Lauren with her niece, Madison Thibault

Since we have been home, my granddaughter Maddie has been like a cling-on with her aunt. She missed her so much and when we talk about Lauren having to go back to the hospital, Maddie gets nervous that we will be gone a long time again. Maddie is five years old and when we were in the hospital in Boston, Maddie came up as much as she and her parents could (which was quite a bit), so Maddie understands the situation in the hospital. To my amazement, she wasn't as scared as I thought she would be. In her eyes, she just wanted to hang with her aunt.

Now that we are home, Maddie has been so happy she can be with Lauren any time. When we were in Boston, my son and daughter-in-law bought their first home and it's just on the next street over from our house, so our family is close. It's the nicest feeling knowing that we can see each other without having to drive. Maddie can just walk over through the yard and she's here. Trust me, there are times when I can just as easily walk her home too.

Going through all this is very difficult most of the time in one aspect: I wish I had my family here. My mom's in Florida and the last time I saw her was last December. It's so hard missing her so much and knowing that she can't come here and I can't go there.

Mom, I miss you and love you very much. There are many times I feel your strength being sent to me, when I feel like I just might lose it. There may be many miles between us but I know in our hearts we are not apart. I'm just going to end this one tonight with "Mom, I love you."

Love,

Lynne

Chapter 18

As the World Goes By…

Tuesday, October 29, 2013

Hi, it's Lauren today.

Sometimes when I sit on the couch waiting for my nurse to take my blood pressure, I look over at my mom ironing. When my eyes go back to the Lifetime movie playing and I stick my arm for my nurse, I think how things used to be just a little over a year ago. As the world goes by right now while we're waiting for that damn call, I just think of when I used to be go….go…go. I'd go to school in Boston then hop in my car and head home to work the weekend away then Monday morning back to school, sliding homework in at any free time I could find. I felt so responsible, like I was working toward something in my life, even as I slowly began to get sicker and sicker.

I still tried to keep up. I never thought I'd miss that busy lifestyle but going on almost a year of not working and actually working with half a heart, I want it back. I asked my boyfriend a stupid question today: "Do you think I'm a loser?" He couldn't believe I would even say that; I'm waiting for my new frigging heart. I thought that this little time off given to me to relax was a good idea and waiting for a call wasn't going to be as hard as all the doctors said ….boy, was I wrong!

Waiting is driving me and my family nuts. I don't mean to complain but this is what it's like to wait for a heart (well, my adventure anyway). It got to the point where I literally asked my doctor if they forgot about me. She laughed and said "No, Lauren."

When we began this journey, they all pointed out that I'm a rare blood type and only weighing 110 lbs puts me at an advantage. Well, where is my damn heart now? I've been waiting since March13th, then I was taken off the list when I had all my surgeries in June and got that nice pressure sore in the back of my damn head causing baldness and a lovely wound.

I'm a just a little grumpy and cry more than a normal 23 year old should because I want to feel like a useful part of society again. Because my heart isn't working to full capacity, I'm tired more than I should be. The part that gets me the most is I feel so emotionally alone!.People my age should NOT be trading their hearts in for new ones. I barely broke this one in yet, LOL.

I just know once the call does come, then comes surgery and recovery and the process I already lived through once. God help me if there are any complications or anything. I was put on this earth to do something great; I don't know what it is yet but I'm not leaving without doing it.

I must say, people have been as wonderful and supportive as they were from Day One to now. This is a learning process. I love the people I've met and the ones I was able to touch with my story and attitude toward this. Mom and I were looking at pictures the other day and we could not believe that we were in the hospital for so long. Looking at how nicely our room was decorated; a big thanks to Auntie Donna.

I really just want to get this heart soon, make that 2 hour nerve-racking drive to Boston and start the next chapter of my

STRENGTH

LOVE,
LAUREN

2am, Waiting for the Special Call Wednesday, October 30, 2013

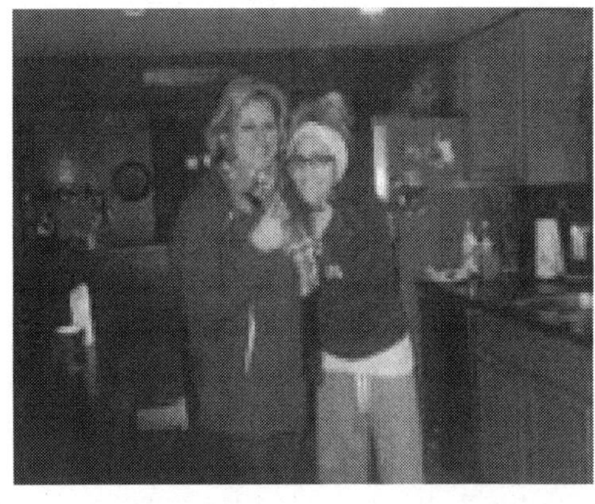

This picture was taken last Thanksgiving. Lauren's favorite night of the year: Black Friday Shopping

Lauren and Kristy McGinn getting ready to hit the stores. My brother Ronnie and his family try to come for Thanksgiving every year (they live in Virginia), so this was Kristy's first time going out on Black Friday. Notice how happy and excited they look. I wish I had a picture of how they looked when they came home in the morning. (Not like this.) They did have a great time and got really good deals, but were very tired. When you look at Lauren, it's hard to tell she was in heart failure, but she was. Her heart at that time was starting to get weaker but that was when she was happy, because her favorite time of the year was starting… Christmas.

If you know Lauren, you know this is when she is the happiest. Lauren loves Christmas. The part she loves the most is giving. At this point, she has most of her Christmas shopping done and wrapped. She has been ordering most online; the UPS and FedEx drivers know us now. When we say she has a big heart, we mean both physically and emotionally. She loves to give and make people feel special. Last year she had more funds to work with as she was working, so this year she has to be more creative in her gift-giving. She told me she that she wants it all done early because we don't know when we will be in the hospital and she doesn't want to worry about it.

The only gift Lauren wants is the gift of life: a new heart. As a mother, you always want to be able to give your kids what they really want for Christmas but this year it is out of my hands. My plan is to make Christmas this year as special as I can, with or without our new heart. Well, it's 2am and I can't sleep. I'm just sitting here looking at the phone, praying it will ring with area code 617. I feel like I have aged so much during this past year. It's so hard to get motivated about anything these days because you never know when we will be back in the hospital. I could get the call right now as I write this post. There are so many times when I feel like it is so hard to just breathe; the stress and anxiety can be very overwhelming at times.

This Saturday will be the end of Lauren's 30 days as a 1A on the transplant list, then she will be a 1B. What that means is we have to submit a petition to get her back as a 1A. So between now and Saturday, if you are saying prayers say them louder and stronger for Lauren PLEASE.
God Bless, Lynne

Part of our prayers were answered
Tuesday, November 5, 2013

Last Saturday Lauren was supposed to be taken off the 1A list status and put in as a 1B for her heart transplant. We couldn't believe it would happen; all our doctors were convinced that she would have gotten the call before this.

Well, we didn't get the call, but we were told by the hospital that they are going to keep her a 1A for two more weeks. Reason being, she is at a high risk for infections. With the LVAD in her heart there is a risk she could get an infection with the device. When she had her defibrillator in her, during her open heart surgery to have the LVAD inserted, her surgeon noticed there was a spot on her heart that didn't

look right. He did a biopsy and it showed she had an infection from one of the defibrillator leads. She then had to undergo another surgery to have the defibrillator removed. Lauren has been, and still is, on antibiotics now to prevent any type of infection. So as of today, she is a 1A; that was a wonderful phone call. I must say, when I saw the 617 area code on my phone, my heart jumped and my hands were shaking, thinking it was a heart. But this news was great.

I was just looking at my band on my wrist and started thinking… Lauren is so blessed that so many wonderful people are wearing them to help support her. When I go out there are times I will see someone wearing the purple band and my heart just melts, thinking so many people care about her. Thank you very much. Just throwing it out there, if anyone would like to purchase one please contact Lauren or myself. They are $5.00 with the proceeds going toward her care.
God Bless
Much love, Lynne

Donate Life, Something to Think About
Friday, November 8, 2013

Have you ever thought about it
If not, it's never too late to sit back and give it some thought

www.donatelife.net

Just Some Thoughts
Monday, November 11, 2013

As I sit here ready to write a new post, my mind keeps racing as to what I would like to write about. The one thing that keeps popping into my mind is Christmas. I keep wondering what our Christmas will be like. Will we be home still waiting, or in the hospital or home with Lauren's new heart?

I've decided I'm going to start decorating for the holiday this week. The one thing no one is going to take away from us is Christmas. If we happen to be in the hospital, when we come home we'll be all set. I'll just do the inside right now; don't want our neighbors thinking we're crazy.

As we sit here waiting for the call, I just want my daughter to smile and have some fun. So all you friends out there give her a call.

Love,
Lynne

Who Makes the Decision About Organ Distribution?
Tuesday, November 12, 2013

UNOS : Donate Life

141

United Network for Organ Sharing

I have been asked quite a few times how Lauren will receive her heart (who decides). Well, I hope this post will help. UNOS is the organization that has all the data from all over the country as to who is waiting for an organ. The data center is located in Richmond, Virginia and it's broken down into eleven geographic regions to enable transplantation. Also, it's broken down by blood type, organ, time waiting and status levels. We live in Region 1, which consists of all of New England.

UNOS is involved in many aspects of the organ transplant and donation process:

- Managing the national transplant waiting list, matching donors to recipients 24 hours a day, 365 days a year.
- Maintaining the database that contains all organ transplant data for every transplant event that occurs in the U.S.
- Bringing members together to develop policies that make the best use of the limited supply of organs and giving all patients a fair chance at receiving the organ they need, regardless of age, sex, ethnicity, lifestyle, or financial/social status.
- Monitoring every organ match to ensure organ allocation policies are followed.
- Providing assistance to patients, family members and friends.
- Educating transplant professionals about their important role in the donation and transplant process.
- Educating the public about the importance of organ donation.

United Network for Organ Sharing (UNOS) is the private, non-profit organization that manages the nation's organ transplant system under contract with the federal government.

To learn more about UNOS, visit www.unos.org

Hope I explained it well,

Lynne

Chapter 19

Memories

Thursday, November 14, 2013

I was looking through some pictures and thought I would like to share some. The last few days, I just keep crying thinking that Lauren will be back in the hospital again. Not sure if I am strong enough to do it again.

I love my daughter so much, it kills me that my child has to go through all of this.

This was taken shortly after being admitted. My sister Donna brought Lauren some snow from outside.

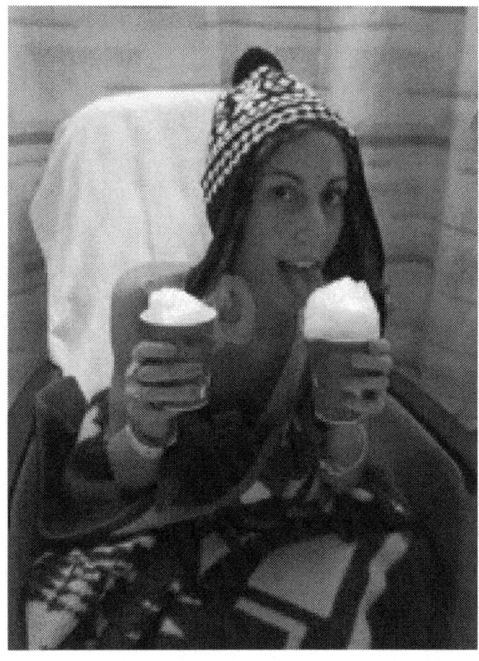

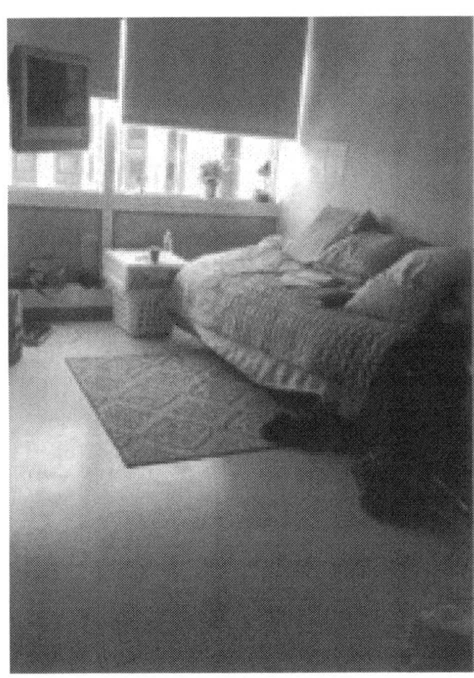

This was my bed in Lauren's hospital room. My sister Donna brought me all the comfy bedding plus a rug.

Lauren with her feeding tube in.

PA line in her neck. My granddaughter called her Stufnufugus.

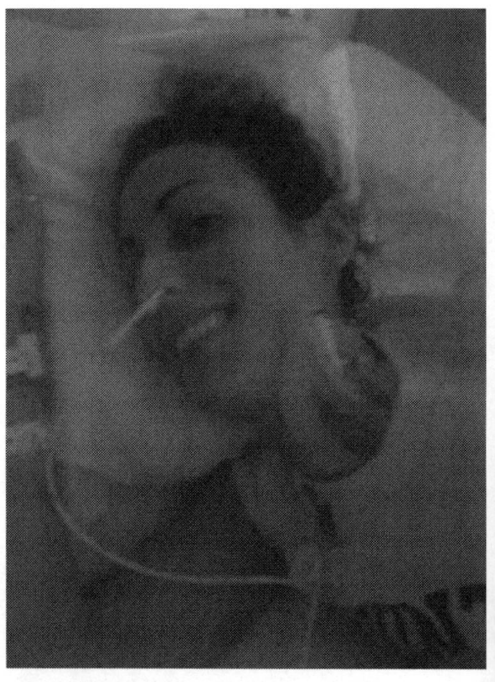

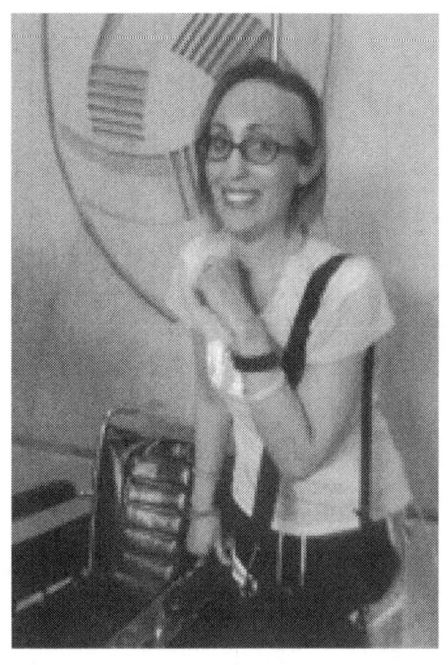

Lauren after our first shopping trip. The black bag is her controller that she needs to carry with her at all times. It is connected right into her heart.

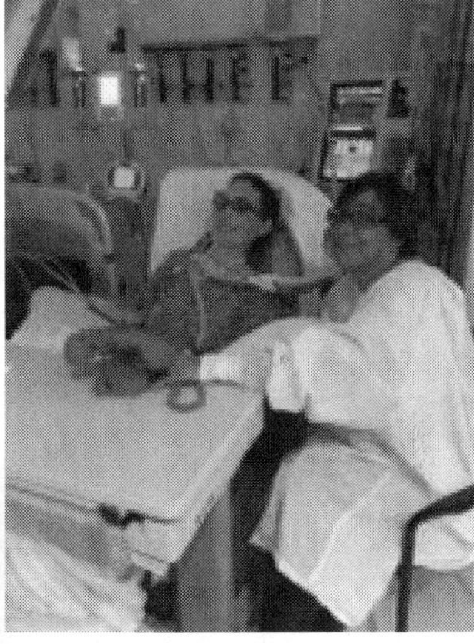

Lauren with her Auntie Donna hanging out.

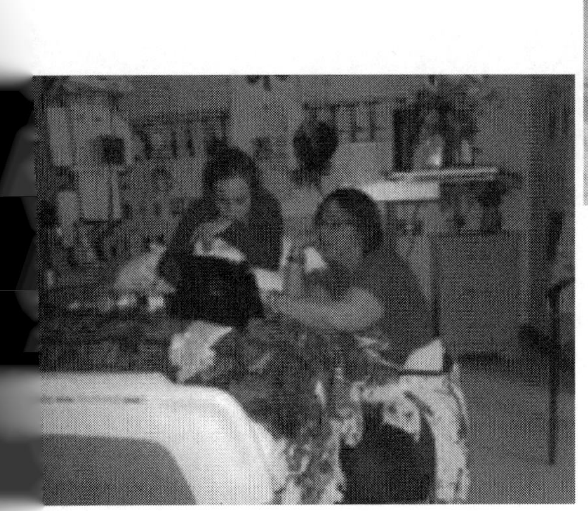

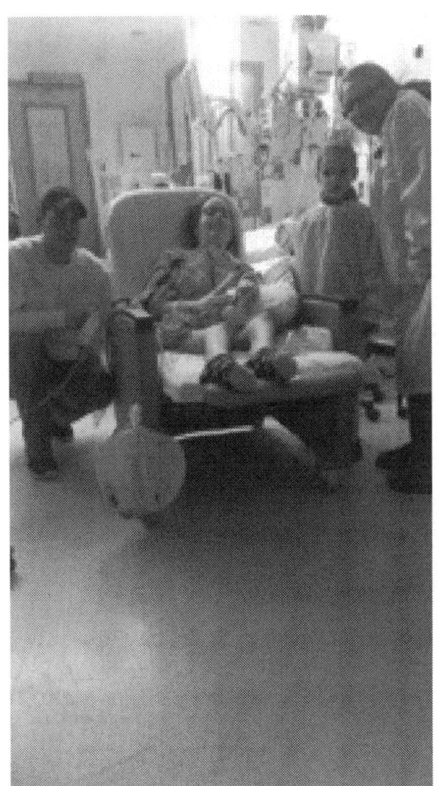

My son Michael, my daughter-in-law Katie and granddaughter Madison, with Lauren.

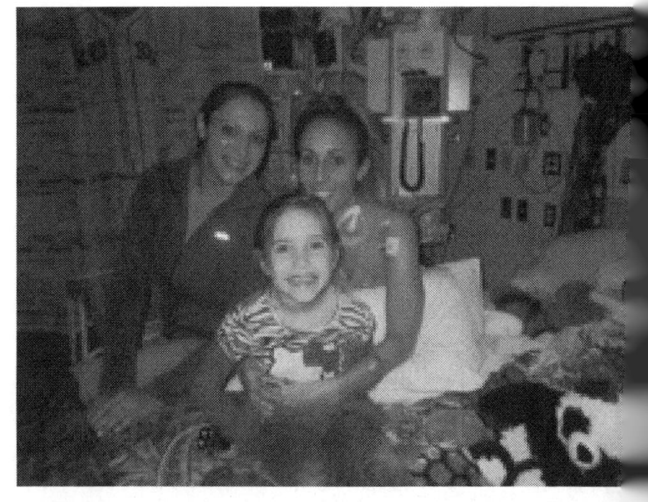

Katie, Lauren and Madison

What a Day!
Wednesday, November 20, 2013

I need to tell you about the day Lauren and I had!
Be ready, you're not going to believe this:
It all started around 7am when Lauren came into my room saying, "Come on, Mom; don't sleep the day way, coffee is on."

As I was sitting downstairs waiting for her to finish with her shower, she came running down the stairs saying she had a big day ahead of her. As she grabbed the keys to her car, she said, "Have a great day, see you later." Seeing her in her car, being the independent woman she has become, what a great way it was to start the day. As the day went on, I called her to ask if she could stop at the store to pick up a few things.

Later on, when Lauren came home, she was so full of life, telling me she had a very productive day, getting things done. I was doing some yard work, so she said, "Here Mom, sit down for a bit, I'll finish mowing the lawn and those weeds aren't going to pull themselves. I'll take care of those while I'm at it, can you just grab me the gloves, please? Don't want to get my freshly-painted nails wrecked." *What a great kid*, was all I was thinking. After we finished the yard work together, Lauren told me she was going out to dinner with a couple of friends, then maybe grab a few drinks and go dancing.

That's what we would call "a perfect day," only one problem: I woke up. A mother's dream. Yes, it was all in a dream. Lauren can't do any of those things now.

I dream about this all the time. I want my daughter back. She used to do these things (okay, except wake up at 7am). If you know her, you know she's not a morning person. I would do anything to have that life back. Being a mom with an active, motivated and independent young woman with goals and dreams. Most of all, to be able to just have fun and enjoy life.

This past year so much was taken away from us and we just want it back with Lauren stronger than ever. We know we will get the call but the waiting is really starting to take a toll on us. It's just been a long year!

I PRAY OUR DREAM COMES TRUE SOON……….

Love,
Lynne & Lauren

Merry Christmas
Friday, December 27, 2013

We may not have received a Christmas heart but we did have a miracle of our own. Lauren is alive and we are home with our family. Lauren was able to play Santa, like she does every year in our house. Our doctors are so surprised she hasn't received her new heart by now, so the only thing I can think is that God has a very special one for her. We had a great Christmas and I did receive some good news: my mother, who lives in Florida, told me yesterday that she is planning a trip to Massachusetts. It has been over a year since I saw her last; that was last December when Lauren and I went down to get away right before she became very sick.

I am no different from anyone else; I need my mother. You know that special hug that only your mother can give you? Love you, Mom.

At this point, we are so ready to say goodbye to 2013,
WELCOME 2014

With much Love, Lynne & Lauren

Chapter 20

617 ON MY PHONE

December 29, 2013

It was a Sunday morning. Like every morning, first thing I do is look at my phone just in case I missed something. Nothing there. I made my coffee and said my prayer, "Dear Lord, please let today be the day," then said the Our Father and Hail Mary.

As I went along the morning doing what I normally do, my phone rang. Taking a look, it was area code 617. I started to shake, yelled to my husband, then answered. On the other end, it was the call we all dreamed about. It was Lauren's transplant doctor. Very quietly and calmly he said, "Hello Lynne, this is Dr. Steward, and yes, this is the cal you've been waiting for. We have a heart for Lauren."

I literally fell to the floor crying; my husband had to take the phone foı a second. I then thought, *Oh my God, Lauren.* We ran upstairs to her bedroom as I yelled, "Lauren get up, get up, Dr. Steward's on the phone and they have a heart!" She looked at me like I had two heads o something before it hit her. I put the phone on speaker and she was able to hear it for herself. It was 10:13am. Dr. Steward told us to pack the car and drive up to the hospital. "How much time do we have?" I asked. He told us to be there for 3pm, that they'd be waiting for us at Admissions.

Next thing I did was call my son Mikey. Since he lives on the next street, I think he was over before I finished telling him. He kept asking me if I wanted him to call the police to get an escort to the hospital since we had a 90 mile drive. I told him no, we had plenty of time to get there. We had our bags packed already but needed to pack our last-minute items. The whole time I could not stop crying; my husband just kept telling me to breathe. My son's best friend Ryan came over to offer his help. I asked him to go upstairs and get Lauren moving.

Lauren was moving around her room trying to think of what she wanted to bring. The only thing she was serious about was her signed soccer ball from Rod Steward. I looked at her and laughed and said "Really? Let's just bring the basics now and whatever you want later, we can bring up to the hospital." She was serious but I wasn't ready to walk around the hospital with a soccer ball while she was in surgery. As Ryan helped Lauren get her shoes on and get down the stairs, my son was helping to pack up the car and I think I was just running around in circles.

I always dreamed of this day; I never knew really how I was going to react. Reality just hit.

Okay, time to go. Lauren got into the back seat, pillow in hand (she likes to be comfortable when she travels). We said our goodbyes and everyone said they would meet us at the hospital. So off we went.

I used to wonder what the car ride would be like. It was very quiet. Lauren actually fell asleep in the back seat. Dean and I did not speak; we were lost in our own thoughts. I kept looking back to take a glance at Lauren, praying for her to survive the operation and for the new heart to be successful.

We arrived at hospital admissions around 2pm and within minutes were told they'd take us to get ready for surgery. I was wondering how long it would be before I'd be in my car again going home with my daughter. Our last hospital stay was six months. Not sure if I can do that again but I will do whatever I need to, to get her back home with us.

With Lauren all settled in, the waiting begins. We were told that her new heart is not at the hospital yet; it's being flown in. Lauren keeps asking the doctor where it's coming from but he's not allowed to relay that information. He said, "If Lauren was having a baby, the baby would be wearing pink and this person is someone Lauren would hang out with." So we gathered it was a female, probably around her age. My thoughts kept returning to this family that is grieving right now at this moment, but I still couldn't wait for the heart to arrive just the same. Talk about messed up feelings.

At this point now our family is all with us.

We figured Lauren's donor must be on life support. Around 7pm they started prepping for her surgery. Reality was now setting in. *Is this going to be the last time I talk with my daughter?* I looked atLauren and wondered what she was thinking.

How scared was she? She never let it out. Then those words, "We're ready, time to take you." In my head I yelled, *NO, NO!* As I watched everyone give Lauren hugs and kisses, tears starting to roll down my face. Everyone had tears and assured her they were happy tears for her new heart.

When it was my time to say goodbyes, I gave her a big hug, kissed her, and told her, "stay strong my little Pollock, I am not going anywhere. When I leave this hospital it will be with you in the back seat of the car with a healthy, strong heart and no machines." Then they took her through the doors to the surgical unit. Once she was out of sight, I just broke down and cried and cried in my husband's arms. Now our wait would really begin…

Chapter 21

Lauren's new heart

December 30, 2013

This is really happening. We were told the surgery would be about 8 hours; we were in for a long evening. Throughout the night I spoke with my family on the phone. It was hard with them living in Florida and Virginia. Dean fell asleep on and off, which I encouraged; no need for both of us to be a mess tomorrow, one of us should be slightly alert. During the evening I cried for Lauren and also for the family of the donor. My child has a chance to live while they are morning a death. I knew in my heart, the new heart Lauren was receiving would be a perfect match. God wouldn't let two beautiful people die tonight.

The surgeon finally came out to speak to Dean and I at 5 am and told us everything was good. I was told that the first heartbeat was at 12:15 am. We were able to see Lauren around 6am. Walking into the room, you can never be prepared for what you may see. So many monitors and machines. Lauren's chest was open (due to swelling); they told us this was normal and they planned on closing it tomorrow. Looking at my daughter lying there with tubes coming out of her chest into machines all around her was the scariest thing I had ever witnessed. I kept reassuring myself, *she's alive, she's alive.*

The rest of the day was filled with phone calls to keep everyone posted. All right, I need to be honest, Dean made most of the calls. I was so tired from being up all night, I ended up passing out from pure

exhaustion. Last night Dean had taken a couple of cat naps so he was okay.
My son came with his family to see his sister. With Lauren being in the ICU, only two people were allowed to be in her room at once so every-one took turns sitting with her. When Mikey was getting ready to leave, he and I went to Lauren's room. As we were standing there, all I kept thinking was how much I love my children.

He gave Lauren a kiss on the cheek and as I was walking him out of the ICU, alarms started to sound. We turned to see doctors and nurses running into Lauren's room. My heart sank, I looked at my son, "Oh my God, not Lauren's room!" We ran. When we reached her room, her nurse was sitting on top of her doing chest compressions. Her heart monitor showed nothing but a flat line. My son grabbed me and I yelled for someone to get Dean.

The next thing I knew, Dean was holding me and the nurses wouldn't let me see what was going on in the room. *My daughter is gone* was all that was going on in my head. In all of the commotion, one of the nurses came out and said "We got her back." At that point, more ma-chines were being brought in, one being an x-ray machine. Her nurse had worked so hard on her that she ended up fracturing one of Lau-ren's ribs.

After what seemed like hours, they were able to get her stable. Once she had been stabilized long enough and the swelling had gone down, then they could consider closing her chest. Now it was time to just sit with her and pray.

Friday, January 3, 2014.

New Year, New Beginnings

Lauren is doing well. The doctors have scheduled the surgery for today to close her chest finally. It has been open about five days now, longer than we all thought. During that time she had a few complications but now she's moving in the right direction. I haven't spoken to her yet; they are keeping her sedated until they close the chest. Lauren's last trip into surgery.

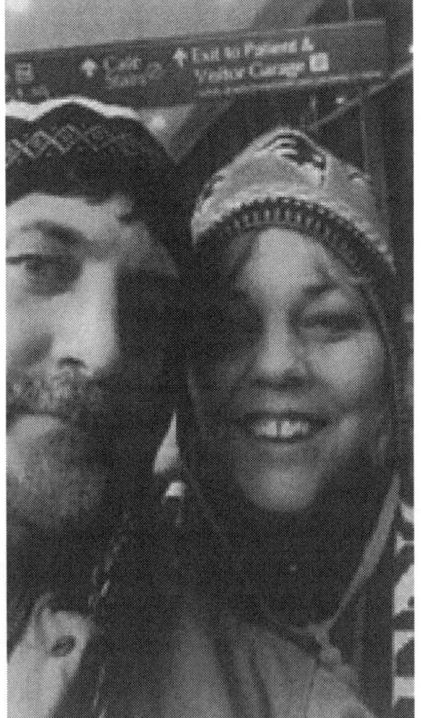

Update

Saturday, January 04, 2014

VERY HAPPY PARENTS

Yesterday Lauren went into surgery to have her chest closed. It was a success! When I saw her afterwards, that was when I realized this was her heart now and it's here to stay. I know it may sound weird, but that was how I felt. All closed in. Lauren is amazing and doing very well. She's not awake yet, still on the breathing machine, but the plan is to take her off on Monday.

Today they are going to lift some of the sedation so she can wake up a bit. I'll finally be able to see those beautiful brown eyes again. If she becomes too irritable due to the breathing tube, they will sedate her enough to be comfortable, but at least we will be able to say hi and comfort her.

The nursing staff here is wonderful; I call them Lauren's Angels. One doctor came in and forgot to put a gown on over his clothes and a nurse stopped him, reminding him to put one on. He rolled his eyes at her and she said, "Don't roll your eyes at me; Lauren is my total priority, no exceptions." I had to laugh.

Love,
Lynne

Monday, January 06, 2014

Today is going to be a very special day. Lauren's breathing tube is going to be removed. Positive thoughts that her lungs will be strong enough to breathe on their own. If not, they will have to perform a tracheotomy.

Yesterday they lifted the sedation a little and we were able to talk to her and see her brown eyes. She actually flashed a smile at me. Obviously she can't speak with the tube, so we were communicating with hand movements. She liked when I gave her a foot massage; when I would stop she would raise her hand for me to keep going. Telling me what to do already…I'd rub her feet all day if she wanted me to; anything for her. I'm really starting to believe she is on the road to recovery.

This morning I couldn't sleep so I went outside; it was about 3:30am and it was raining. To me, that was a good sign. The first time Lauren went outside when we were in the hospital before, it was raining. I remember the look on her face having the rain fall down on her. She told me it was the best feeling in the world. Also, the day we left the hospital on August 23, 2013, it was raining. So today it is a big day for her and it's raining.

Love,
Lynne

Chapter 22

Recovery Begins

January 7, 2014

For most people, recovery would be 4 weeks (tops) for a heart transplant. But I can almost guarantee this is not going to be our case. Lauren's muscle disease plays a big factor in her recovery. Her muscles get very weak and it may take much longer for her to regain her strength. Not only her muscles, but her lung functions have become very weak too. I'm prepared to stay for a while. Every night I pray that this is not the case. I'm not sure how I can stay in the hospital for another lengthy period of time but we've come this far and this is the finish line.

Like the little engine said, "I think I can, I think I can."

On the Road to Recovery

Thursday, January 09, 2014

I'm so happy to say Lauren is on the road to recovery. It was quite bumpy early on, but as of this morning things look like they may go her way. Yesterday she had to have a tracheotomy performed and they did it right in her room because they didn't want to move her; too many machines are attached to her.

On Tuesday, they tried to extubatne (remove the breathing tube), but she lasted only a short time on her own and the doctors had to place it back in. Very upsetting. I just keep wondering why things just can't go smooth for her. Well, we have been down this road before with the tracheotomy tube. At least now she won't have to be sedated; she'll be able to sit up and maybe tomorrow we can start moving forward like trying to stand. I feel like I can breathe a little easier.

Yesterday the nurses kept asking me if I was okay; they even had the social worker come to sit with me. Dean kept telling me I didn't look right. With Lauren now awake, she wants me with her at all times. At times, it's very frustrating not knowing what she may need. It catches up with me. Pure exhaustion. I've just been numb; we've had too many ups and downs and I feel like I just don't have any emotion left in me. My phone rings and I just give it to Dean; I'm not even in the mood to talk. Again I sit here and watch Lauren's heart rate monitor as if it's a TV, making sure it stays stable.

After the tracheotomy was done, Dean and I looked at Lauren. We can now see her beautiful face without tubes and tape. She is so much more comfortable. I was totally exhausted so Dean took the first shift sitting with her and holding her hand so I could get some rest in order to take the next shift. Lauren just wanted one of us with her.

Since she can't talk, we played the game of lip-reading and using a letter board to help us communicate with each other this morning. This is funny: Lauren asked where her battery pack is; I just giggled and told her she doesn't have it any more. She gave me the biggest smile.

The other night Dean and I were sitting in the chapel and I met a lovely woman. I asked her how her patient was doing and she told me she comes to pray for all the patients here. We sat and talked about Lauren and she told me she would say extra prayers for her.

At this moment, Lauren's numbers look good, her breathing looks good and even her spirits are up. We are going to be here for a while, but that's okay. I know we'll make it home and she'll be a brand new person (NO HEART FAILURE).

Today is going to be Lauren's first biopsy. They check to make sure her heart likes its new home.

Love,
Lynne, Dean & Lauren

Sitting Up
Saturday, January 11, 2014

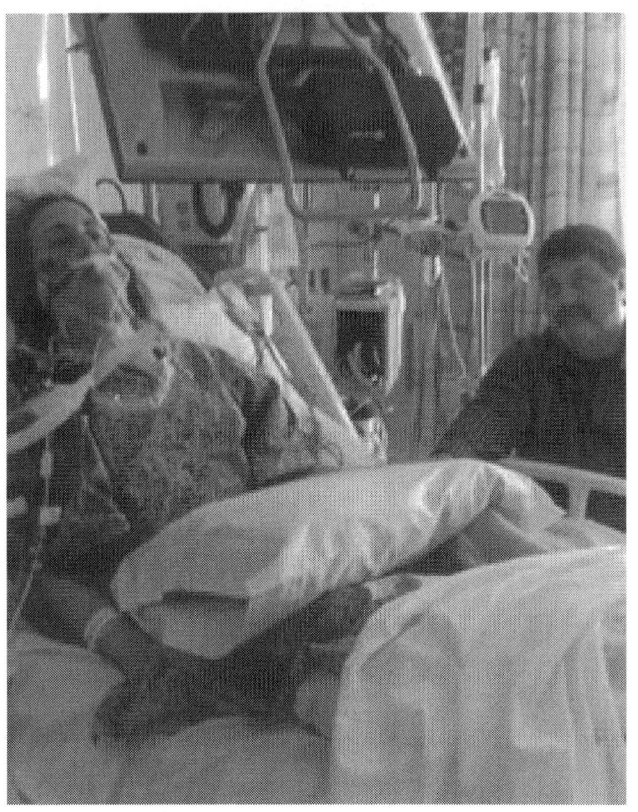

Lauren sat up for the first time today; a very happy moment. When they sat her up they did it just for a bit, not wanting to exert her or her new heart too much. It was a beautiful sight.

The results from her biopsy came back negative, meaning her body likes her new heart. No rejection. Great news! She will have another one next week; they need to keep testing it.

Lauren has been on so many medications that have kept her sedated that now that they have stopped them, she is having a hard time remembering what has happened to her. We just need to keep telling her that she received her new heart.

have so many thoughts that I would like to pass on but my mind is too fuzzy. The other day I was so nervous that I actually gave myself a bruise on my arm from holding it so tight for so long. It's going to be a longer recovery than we thought but we'll do what we need to do.

Okay, here's a good one: If you know Lauren, you know her favorite pastime is sleeping. Well, the last two days she has not slept, not even a nap. I tell the nurses this is NOT my daughter. The new heart is working so well she's not tired at all. Finally, today she is getting a little rest. The doctors explained to Dean and I that it's all the meds (and she is also on steroids). Can't wait until she is finally coherent to tell her she wouldn't sleep.

Love,

Lynne

Wednesday, January 15, 2014

Sorry I haven't updated; I know everyone is concerned. Lauren is still in ICU on the breathing machine with her trache. Her lungs are not quite strong enough to breathe on their own just yet. The doctors have been concerned and ordered a chest x-ray. She has some fluid in her lungs at this point. Not good; could be very dangerous for her. I will keep everyone posted when I know more.

She has a long road ahead of her but I keep telling her we are one step closer to going home. Her heart is working beautifully and we're now

just dealing with complications after the surgery. These problems basically arose from when she flat-lined. All organs take a hit when the heart stops. Keep the prayers coming, we need them.
Love, Lynne & Dean

Second Biopsy
Thursday, January 16, 2014

Lauren is having a second biopsy on her heart today. We won't get the results until tomorrow. My poor daughter has been through hell and back. Her first biopsy came back great, so the doctors told me this morning that they feel very positive about this one. At this point, it's hard for me to put into words everything that has been happening, but down the road I will.

What I can say is, she's in the right place with excellent doctors and nurses. Dean had to go back to work so my sister Donna is here with us. If you text me and I don't answer, I'm sorry, I'm focused on Lauren.

I feel like this is a roller coaster ride; so many ups and downs. Lauren and I *are* going to walk out of this hospital someday. (I made a doctor promise me that, I needed to hear it.) It's just going to be a little longer than we thought. The focus at this time is to get her off the respirator. Once that is done we will be on our way. Lungs are still weak. She overcame that before and she'll do it again. I told her, "we just need to work a little harder," she looked at me with a frown and I told her "don't look at me that way, we are fighters and don't give up."

Biopsy results

Friday, January 17, 2014

Second biopsy came back negative, no rejection…
GREAT NEWS!

Nothing Stops Lauren
Saturday, January 18, 2014

I was looking at some pictures this morning and came across one of Lauren parasailing in Florida a few years ago. She is so amazing, nothing stops her from trying something once. This is something I wouldn't even consider doing myself, but not my Lauren.

Now with her new heart there will be no stopping her. I remember going to the gym with her and she would push me; the next day I couldn't even cough, it would hurt so much. That's where I want to be again. And we will be.

At this point in her recovery, they put her vent on pressure support; that is good; it means that they are working her lungs to build them back up. She sat on the side of the bed yesterday with physical therapy for ten minutes; every day a little longer.

Today's plan is to wash her hair. Lauren was talking (she can't talk, I have to read her lips) about her homecoming party. This is funny: she says she wants to have a keg of beer there. I just laughed at her and said, "That's what's on your mind?"

Lauren hates beer.

I told her she could have anything she wants.

Miss everyone back home, Lauren

Lauren Sitting Up for the First Time
Sunday,

Januuary 19,

2014

Finally, we were able to get Lauren to sit up in chair for the first time: BIG MOMENT. She was very nervous so I was holding her hands to tell her she was safe and to calm her. By the expression on her face, sh wasn't happy but I would not let her give up. She got over it and we sa there watching TV for about an hour. The really frustrating part is when she's trying to say something and if I can't make it out by readin her lips, she gets mad. I tell her slow down, then she makes this face at me, like I'm an idiot.

Doctors reported today that they are lowering her vent to eleven. Every day they keep going down, which is great news. Lungs are getting stronger; baby steps. I was standing there when they did the rounds and this is how the doctor started, "Our patient is Lauren Meizo and aside from having a very over-protective mother…" We all laughed.

Today we are going to decorate her room with Patriots balloons to watch the game together. The nurses said she can have balloons in the room.

Love,
Lynne

Snow Heart
Wednesday, January 22, 2014

My sister Donna and I went outside and she made a heart out of snow on the sidewalk last night. The crew that was clearing the walkway shoveled around it, to make it stand out. We wanted to make some snow angels but thought people would look at us funny. We thought a couple of snow angels around the hospital would be appropriate, but to tell you the truth, it was too cold.

Lauren had a good day, she is starting to move her legs and arms a little. I told her she was in Lynne's Boot Camp now. I gave her a ball and she was able to throw it to me. When I threw it back to her into her lap, I would make her pick it up by herself. Also, when she sits in the chair and wants to be reclined, I tell her she has to give me five leg lifts on each leg. The doctors are impressed with her muscle improvement.

Her lungs have been staying clear and she is starting to get less support on the vent. She keeps telling me she's hungry but she can't eat with the respirator. Every day I remind her we are one day closer to walking out the door. If I was to make a guess, I would say maybe by March.

Today is Day 25 since the surgery. When I say March, it feels like a long time, but as long as Lauren is safe and improving each day, it doesn't matter how long it takes. The ICU here on the 6th floor has a wonderful nursing staff, which makes the difference. Very caring, compassionate, and professional staff. I am staying in Lauren's room with her and they have a couch I sleep on. It just makes me feel comfortable knowing I am close to her if she needs anything just in case the nurse isn't in the room at the time. It is a scary place to be with all the machines beeping, it keeps me jumping. I'm getting pretty good at reading them and knowing if Lauren is in trouble. The last couple of days they all have been looking right where they should be for her.

My sister Donna has been here with us, she has a lovely couch in th family room. Then on the weekends, Dean comes and he gets to sleep in a recliner. It is what it is. I'm not complaining at all. I'd sleep on the floor if I had to, you adjust to the situation. I know it's not forever.

Day 30 Since the Transplant
Wednesday, January 29 2014

Well, it's been 30 days today since Lauren received her gift. I finally said enough with the hospital gowns and put one of her shirts on her today. I just cut the back and slipped it on, feels like a million bucks. She looks like herself and it made her feel better.Yesterday the Right IV was taken out of her neck and there was a Hickman Line put into her chest. She needed to have this done. When they need to draw blood, they won't have to be constantly sticking her all the time. It is so great to see all the tubes out of her neck. It was a long day yesterday; she was supposed to have this done at 4pm, but never went into the OR until 10pm. She kept getting bumped for emergencies. She was nervous all day, as was I. All is good today, she looks beautiful.

So the plan for today is for me to wash her hair, give her a good massage, then physical therapy. Tomorrow is going to be her fourth biopsy; send prayers that it comes back negative again. We won't know the results until Friday.

More worrying, that means more wrinkle cream (haha).

Love,
Lynne

Tuesday, February 3, 2014

Update: still in ICU but getting stronger every day. Yesterday, physical therapy came and I suggested the bike pedals so she can work her legs. They brought it in but told me that she's not ready for it yet, maybe in a couple of days. Well, last night I asked her if she wanted to try it and she said yes. I put her feet in the pedals and turned them for her, then she took over and did it herself. I was so excited, like a proud mom watching her child ride a bike by herself for the first time. I ran out of the room to get her nurse to show her, two nurses came in and we all could not stop smiling and Lauren felt great.

Moving forward…yes, they are the professionals but I knew Lauren could do it with a little motivation. I remembered the times we went to the gym together and she would work me until my stomach hurt; that's how we're there for each other.

Love,
Lynne & Lauren

Happy Birthday to a Wonderful Husband & Father
Wednesday, February 05, 2014

It's Dean's birthday today. Lauren and I would like to say "We love you very much and are so very lucky to have you in our lives. You are our rock."

The day I married you and you became my husband and Lauren's father, the gods were smiling down on us. We love you very much. With everything that is going on, it's such a comfort to know we have you to come home to. Happy Birthday!

Lauren's update: Lauren sent her first Facebook message yesterday, typing it herself. We take this type of action for granted but this was a big day in our lives. OMG, she also went on her favorite website and did some shopping, buying a cute shirt. That's my girl. One of the things she really wants to do is get in a wheelchair to get out of this room and take a stroll around the floor. The doctors said that might be possible in a few days.

With the snow coming down today it will look pretty for her to see. There is a big window by the elevators that goes from floor to ceiling with a beautiful view. You can see for miles; that's where I dream of taking her to see the outdoors.

She has had four biopsies so far. The first three came back negative (no rejection), but the one last week came back with a slight rejection. The doctors told Dean and I it is common but it wasn't the news we wanted to hear. She is scheduled for another biopsy this Thursday. With the rejection, they need to increase her anti-rejection medication. With that said, this medication makes her weak so she has to work harder to keep moving forward.

Love,
Lynne & Lauren

First time out of her room

Friday, February 07, 2013

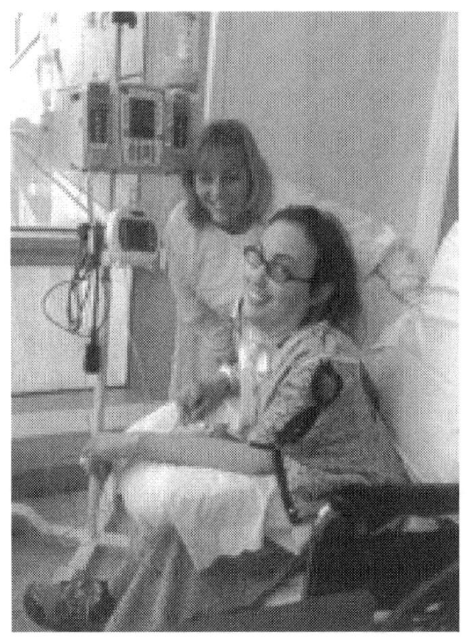

One of Lauren's requests has been to go in a wheelchair and take a stroll around the unit. Well, her day finally arrived! When the doctors told us the news, we looked at each other like two little kids about to do something forbidden. You know that look. But we have permission. So many times, Lauren and I would talk about just doing it but we knew we couldn't. Now we can! In my head, I said, *check, one step closer to going home.*

They have been weaning Lauren off the ventilator and now she is on a trache collar. When PT came in they brought a wheelchair and said "Let's get out of here." Lauren was so happy and very nervous. The therapists told us she is making great strides and we have been doing our homework faithfully every day, working her muscles. There have been many times when she didn't want to do her exercises but I wouldn't let her slide.

When we took our walk, there were five of us. A nurse, three physical therapists and of course, Mom. Lauren felt like a celebrity, the nurses and the doctors on the floor were so amazed to see her out of her room. Our walk led us to the elevators where the big window is. It was like a magical moment when Lauren saw the outside world for the first time. Tears were starting to grow (okay, all around) and I asked if she was okay. Lauren answered, "I really didn't think I would see the outdoors ever again."

"I knew you would." I assured. We just sat there looking at the snow coming down. It was a beautiful time. Lauren had the biggest smile on her face, all I can say is that it was priceless.

Today she is having her fifth biopsy. Normally she wouldn't have one this week but with the last one, the doctors want to check it again. So again, the waiting game begins. We don't get the results until tomorrow.

She's getting stronger but she tells me she doesn't see it. I have to keep reminding her that everyone else sees it.

> Visitors are welcome, I'm sure she is getting tired of me. If you would like to visit, let me know (no flowers, ICU rules)

Love, Lynne

Great News Update
Saturday, February 8, 2014

Yesterday was a dream day. I thought I was dreaming. Good news all day and I'm so happy Dean was here with us. He normally comes on Friday after work but he surprised us Thursday evening.

Lauren's biopsy came back negative, no rejection!

Her doctors told us that all her pressures are normal and the left and right side of her heart are working strong. The fluid she had around the heart is gone. The doctors gave me a hug and said "she's doing great." It meant so much to me. I find myself telling Lauren her gift must have come from an athlete, nice and strong.

Also, they changed her trache to a smaller one, then they gave her a speaking valve so she spoke for the first time. She looked at Dean and said "I love you, Dad." She kept the speaking valve in for just a short time in order to not work herself too hard.

With Lauren in her wheelchair, we took two walks around the unit. PT has been working with her, having her use her arm to wheel the chair then with her feet to move the chair a bit. Monday she is scheduled for a swallow test and if all goes well she will finally be able to eat and drink. She's told me the first thing she wants is a fruit salad.

You know how when everything is finally going in the right direction, you keep holding your breath, just waiting for someone to pull the rug out from under you? No one pulled our rug out.

Love,
Lynne & Lauren

Very confusing?

Tuesday, February 11, 2014

Lauren was going to have a speech and swallow test today but it didn't happen. Her schedule is such that she's supposed to be up every day by 10am but she was tired and she didn't get up until noon. At that point, the speech and swallow therapist came in to do the test and she was just not waking up so the test didn't happen. I asked if she could come back later and was told she will be back tomorrow. I was so upset; to me, tomorrow just means another day of waiting and sitting around.

The part that is so confusing to me is some nurses tell me I have to speak up and get her moving in the morning, then other nurses say she needs her rest so they give her some meds and then she sleeps. I'm trying so hard to help her without stepping on toes but I know my daughter. At this point in her recovery, she really needs to be pushed. I'm not here to make friends, but I do live here.

This morning I woke up at 2am and noticed Lauren was sound asleep still in her chair. I looked for a nurse and couldn't find one so I laid back down. I fell asleep, then woke up around 5am and they had just finished putting her to bed. WTF? Just so frustrating. I hate living in the hospital. It seems like no one is on the same page; different nurses, different doctors all the time and they all have their own opinions.

Lynne

Friday, February 14, 2014

It's been a couple of days since I updated. I know everyone is concerned, I just haven't been able to get my thoughts together. It's been a hell of a week. Lauren was supposed to be moved out of ICU on Monday but it's Friday and we're still here. One of the reasons was there was not a bed available. Then she had some fluid building up on the outside of her right lung (this has been going on for a while) and the doctors thought her body would just absorb it. Well, it didn't.

On Wednesday we were in her room with PT working on getting her to stand when out of nowhere, she couldn't breathe. I ran out into the hallway and yelled for help, with the doctors and nurses rushing in. She had a blockage in her tracheotomy tube so they needed to change it. This is a sight no parent should ever have to see; her lips were blue with terror in her eyes. After that episode, they took an ultrasound of her chest and found the fluid was constricting her right lung.

Yesterday the doctors placed what is called a "pig tail" in her to drain the fluid. The procedure was done in her room; it was set up like a mini operating room. During the procedure they went through her back on the right side and inserted a tube where the fluid was. They left the tube inside her to drain the fluid. When they did it, a liter of fluid came out right away. I was told that her right lung was almost folded because her chest was so full. So with that said, I was so thankful she'll now be able to breathe better. She told me she felt sore and the doctors said it will take a while for her lung to expand to where it should be.

Last night Lauren felt like she should cap her trache and the nurse agreed. Capping the trache means just what it sounds like. We cap her trache hole so no air goes through the opening. When the cap in this means she's doing all the breathing through her nose and mouth. During that time she was doing great. It was so nice to sit with her and talk.

As we were sitting there watching TV, she fell asleep so I went to the kitchenette down the hall to make myself a cup of tea. When I returned, I noticed that the heart monitor showed her heart rate was up a little so I went over to the chair to check her. She looked flushed and bubbles were coming out of her mouth. I suctioned her mouth and kept calling her name but she was unresponsive. I hit the call button but was told the nurse was busy and would be in soon. I ran out into the hallway and yelled "SHE'S UNRESPONSIVE, HELP!" Boy, did I get the whole floor in her room fast!

Lauren was unconscious and they had to bag her to wake her up. Turns out she was not letting enough air be expelled, breathing on her own, and carbon monoxide was building up. The doctors checked her trach and there was no blockage; she just needed to breathe with deep breaths. After that, I had to work on keeping her awake to make sure she was responsive. This went on for about an hour, then she seemed fine. There is talk about maybe putting her back on the respirator but please pray this does not happen.

As I'm writing this, so many thoughts are going through my head. I pray my daughter will get that strength she needs to overcome everything that is happening to her.

Love,
Lynne

Chapter 23

Out of ICU Again
Wednesday, February 19, 2014

Yesterday they told us we were moving to step down, didn't want to say anything until we really did. It couldn't have happened at a better time; I was really starting to lose it. Living in ICU for 2 months takes a toll on you, especially your frame of mind. A couple of days ago, I just prayed that Lauren would get stronger. I really couldn't take any more, I was starting to feel like I was losing the strength to keep going. As of Monday, it has been 8 weeks since the surgery, so this is 8 weeks we can put behind us and keep moving forward.

The other day Lauren was just kinda being a tad bit lazy. At this point in her recovery we need to keep moving with her PT and it will help with getting her lungs stronger. I had a talk with one of her doctors and she told me I have to keep pushing her; the only person that is going to make Lauren stronger is Lauren. I expressed to her how when there are times I try to push her a little (now I am talking just sitting in a wheelchair) to help strengthen her core muscles, I get looks from the nurses, then they ask Lauren if she wants to do it, she'll say no, so they won't push it. Guess who looks like the bad guy?

I want to go home someday so I told Lauren she's going to have to work to make it happen. I wasn't fooling around, so we got in the chair, visited a couple of patients and I made her do some physical therapy in the chair, like trying to push it a little with her arms and then take a few steps. She wasn't happy with me but I said, "Hate me today, you'll love me tomorrow." That evening Lauren told me she loved me for pushing her.

Love,
Lynne

P.S. Here is a funny thing I saw tonight: The escalator was not working to go down, so I just walked down the stairs. Two nurses stood there and said "Oh no, we'll have to take the elevator" and they did. I couldn't help but laugh.

Tuesday, February 25, 2014

Last Friday was a great day. Lauren had her swallow test and passed. She can eat and drink finally. Soft foods to start with. The biopsy came back negative (no rejection) and her cathode came out. Moving forward…

She has graduated; doesn't have to have her next biopsy until next month. At this point, she still needs to work hard on building her mus cles up and improving her breathing. Yesterday in the conversation the word ***HOME*** was involved. We will probably be here two or three more weeks, depending on Lauren, and then a rehab hospital for a bit

Every day is so different. Yesterday she didn't feel well at all. The meds that she has to take now upset her stomach, so after she got her meds yesterday she threw up. Her stomach was upset all day so no physical work could be done. The doctors are trying to find the proper mix of meds. I hope today will be one of the good days.

Love,
Lynne

Thursday, March 6, 2014

I know I need to update; so many thoughts and well, to sum it up, Lauren is back in ICU. Last week everything seemed to be going great, moving forward. They were getting us ready to go to a rehab hospital. I couldn't believe this was finally happening. We were having meetings with the pharmacist regarding proper doses and med times. I couldn't stop smiling, we were finally in the "we are going home" mode. I know it will be a couple of weeks but the end is getting closer.

With everything that has been happening, Lauren has been experiencing high anxiety. After being a patient for so long, I can say we are both nervous.

Last Friday she was having a lot of anxiety and the doctors tried a new drug on her. This medication made her breathing very shallow, which resulted in not allowing her to release enough carbon dioxide. Before I knew it, she was back in the ICU. We were lucky they noticed it right away. Needless to say, she can't use that drug. Since her surgery, the meds that she was taking for anxiety can't be taken now.

We have been practicing different relaxation exercises plus therapy. Yesterday the doctor took out her trache and she is doing great without it. It has been capped for a week but to be on the safe side they did not want to remove it sooner. Having it out makes us feel a little closer to the door to leave.

As a mother, I just want to take away her anxiety and take care of her with love and hugs. Yes, I can do that to a point but she is 23 with fears none of us could ever imagine.

The other day I was walking toward her room when one of her doctors stopped and told me I look like shit. They asked if I was feeling okay, then told me I need to go home for a bit. I told them I wan't leaving my daughter here alone.

We were in Lauren's room and I coughed; the doctor snapped, "Are you sick?" Then went on to explain how important it is that Lauren not be near anyone that is ill. I told them I feel fine and am taking my vitamins. I told Dean what the doctors said and he told me he'd stay with her so I could leave. I wouldn't be able to go home and sit there alone. I want to be with my family. The only time I can spend time with Dean is when he comes here to the hospital; that is our family time.

Love,
Lynne

Tuesday, March 11, 2014

LAUREN IS OUT OF ICU…
AGAIN

We got our wish.

Lauren is getting stronger and they are in the process of making arrangements for rehab, maybe by the end of the week.

PLEASE LORD, KEEP US ON THIS TRACK

Love,
Lynne

Thursday, March 13, 2014

A year ago on this date, Lauren was officially placed on the heart transplant list. I still remember when the doctors came into the room. Lauren, Dean and I were sitting just waiting for the word. There could be a chance my daughter would live. We knew this would be Lauren's only chance at living a normal life again before all this happened. What most people don't know is that you have to be approved to be placed on a transplant list. Just because you may need a new heart to live, doesn't mean it's easy. So much is involved. A new heart is such a precious gift, they need to know that the recipient is going to take care of it, has the proper support, emotionally, physically and financially (for the meds you will need to take the rest of your life).

At the beginning of our journey, the doctors told us this is not a sprint, it's a marathon. Well, one year later, Lauren has her new heart and today we were supposed to leave the hospital to go to a rehab facility. Because of all the coordination involved, it will be another day.

As I'm sitting here looking out the window, I can't believe it's been a year. Some days it feels like a lifetime. We are getting closer to going home and living our lives as a family again.

Much love always,
Lynne

Friday, March 14, 2014

Remember how I said we were leaving the hospital today? Forget that. Lauren has not been feeling well, throwing up all day. The doctors are trying to figure out what is going on. I told them she is not going to rehab until she is 100%.

Lynne

Out of the Hospital
Thursday, March 20, 2014

Good morning and happy first day of spring.

We finally made it to the rehab hospital. It's been a very emotional day. Happy and sad. Lauren and I were transported by ambulance to the rehab facility. We're getting used to our new environment. The motto here is "Find your strength."

More to come,
Lynne

Chapter 24

Ambulance Ride of a Lifetime

Out of Rehab and Back in the Hospital

Thursday, March 27, 2014

For a short period of time I really thought things were finally going our way. We were in the rehab hospital for only five short days. During our stay there, they made accommodations for me to stay with Lauren in her room. Her room was very small to start with but they gave me a small cot to sleep on. I didn't care; I've slept on worse in the past year and a half. Things seemed to be going well. Lauren was doing her therapy and she liked it here so all was good. Then things changed.

We were sleeping and I heard a nurse in the room putting oxygen on Lauren. I asked what was going on. She said her oxygen stats were going down a bit. I knew what this meant. I was asking Lauren how she felt; I knew this wasn't good. The rest of the evening I stayed up and just watched her, specifically, the way she was breathing. I can differentiate her breathing now.

The following morning she still was not feeling well.. I called the nurse and told her Lauren didn't look good and looked kinda out of it. The nurse suggested that she was probably just tired from last night.

As the morning went on, Lauren still was in and out. She would talk with me then just fall asleep; I knew something was wrong. I called for the doctor and told her we needed a blood gas preformed. I knew the look; been through it a couple of times already. She explained she would call her transplant team to see what they wanted to do.

During that waiting period Lauren was becoming unresponsive. I was very scared. I yelled out for help and the doctor came in and ordered the blood gas.

Results: Lauren was in trouble.

Brigham's was called and was expecting us. The ambulance arrived and as EMTs were quickly getting Lauren for transport, they had to bag her with forced oxygen. She wasn't releasing the carbon dioxide and was in real trouble. As they loaded her into the ambulance, I was told I had to ride in the front seat because they had two EMTs working on her. I was so scared, I didn't think she was going to make it.

When the driver got into his seat he told me to buckle up and hang on. Driving in Boston is an experience in itself but in an ambulance with the lights and the sirens going was totally new to me. We were going down roads the wrong way, making cars move to clear a path for us. I have the utmost respect for all EMTs; they really put their own lives on the line to save others. (I've now experienced that first hand.)

Arriving at the hospital, the staff was waiting for us right at the door. Shit, they were running. They put her into an exam room to assess what was happening, putting her on a bi-pap machine to help with her carbon dioxide level.

In the meantime I called Dean. He was at work but assured me he'd be here as soon as possible. Bi-pap was not working so they informed me that they might have to intubate. I pleaded, "No, please don't." I didn't want to see her on a breathing machine, I just couldn't. Yesterday she was sitting up doing her hair and make-up feeling good. Now today she's going to be alive because of a machine. What the hell is happening?

End result: they needed to insert a breathing tube and Lauren is sedated. She has no idea what is happening to her. The last thing she'll remember is being in the rehab hospital. Dean and I were told she's retaining fluids around her lungs which is making it difficult for her to breathe. My only comfort is that she's with her transplant team. I know they will take great care of my daughter.

Love,
Lynne

Sunday, March 30, 2014

Life back in the ICU.

Lauren still has the breathing tube. She had surgery on Friday to have a Pleurx Catheter inserted. This catheter helps to drain fluids that build up. It will stay in and right now they have it capped; the fluids have drained but having the catheter in will help if the fluids retention reoccurs.

The breathing tube will be removed tomorrow in the Operating Room. Reason being, if there's a problem, she will be in an appropriate environment if they need to do a tracheotomy.

Everyone keeps telling Dean and I that this is just a bump in the road. I'm tired of bumps and I can speak for Lauren when I say she is too.

Gloomy, rainy day today.

They are keeping Lauren lightly sedated to keep her relaxed.
I wish I could get some.

Lynne

Life in ICU
Friday, April 4, 2014

I can't believe it's April already. Lauren received her new heart on December 30. We have hit every bump that could come our way. So as I am writing this, I find it unbelievable we are in ICU. It seems like all the hard work she's done in the last four months never happened.

Unfortunately she did have to have the trache put back in. The doctors told Dean and I that they wanted to put it back in for safety reasons. If she was to build carbon dioxide up again, with difficult breathing, they could just connect the oxygen to the trache. She has a very difficult airway, plus with having the breathing tube in again, her airway has been irritated enough. They had to get a specialist to do the procedure and it had to be performed in the Operating Room.

When she woke up, she was so upset to discover she had a trache again. She was very confused as to why she was back at Brigham's Hospital. We had to explain how she was rushed by ambulance and had been on a ventilator for a week. After hearing what had happened, she just laid back and cried.

Living here is so hard. I've been living here for over a year now and I know all the rules. I have stated this before: my day depends on who Lauren's nurse is. Some nurses are very compassionate, caring, and understanding of our situation. Then we have some nurses that, well, let me just say, aren't.

Done with ICU.

Need to exhale.

Love, Lynne

Tuesday April 8, 2014

Well it finally happened… OUT OF ICU!

We are back on the floor where it all started last March. I think we've been on every floor of this hospital, so I guess it seems appropriate that we leave from where we started. And yes, I did say "leave."

After our last episode at the rehab facility, I told the doctors that when Lauren is ready to go home we are going home, no rehab. That's not just me saying that either.

So anyway, last Friday Lauren's doctor came in to check on her. He said he understands how I feel about going back to a rehab and he agreed. He also told us that Lauren could go HOME! He went on to tell me he's confident I'll take great care of her, along with home nursing and physical therapy.

It was the most incredible news I have heard in a long time.

Our goal is May 1st. My granddaughter's birthday is that day and her party will be on the 3rd. (Lauren missed it last year.)
She has some work ahead of her but she is motivated to make it happen. I love seeing the spark back in her. Yesterday she yelled, "I WANT TO GO HOME!"

Love,
Lynne

Chapter 25

Preparing for the H Word (HOME)

Friday April 11, 2014

The other day the doctors came into Lauren's room and said "We think you'll be able to go home in about two weeks as long as everything keeps moving in the right direction."

I'm still in shock, thinking I'd never hear those words. The doctors told her, "your mother said she's not leaving until she has her daughter with her and she is true to her word."

It's time to have a life outside of the hospital.

I love my daughter so much; she has gone through things a mother would never want to see. Now what I want to see is a smile.

To celebrate the great news, Lauren and I went to the gift shop for a little retail therapy.

Love,
Lynne & Lauren

Be Thankful for Life
Wednesday, April 16, 2014

On Monday Lauren had her eighth biopsy.
Results: negative.
Beautiful news.

The doctors picked a perfect heart for Lauren. I still find it hard to believe it has been four months already. My daughter has overcome every obstacle that could be thrown at her.

As a mother sitting here watching everything that she has gone through, I would never ever wish this on anyone. There are so many times I have to tell myself to keep it together because she needs me.

At this point, everything has been looking good. Her only hurdles now are her breathing and body strength. She still has her trache in and with it being her third one, they are being very cautious. Three tracheotomies in one year could be damaging to vocal cords and her throat anatomy. She has a wonderful otolaryngologist, a doctor that specializes in ear, nose and throat. She told us Lauren doesn't have any damage to her vocal cords but does have some swelling. The plan is to cap the trache today.

As in the past, capping means she will have to breathe from her nose and mouth. If she can support her breathing on her own for a day, they are going to do a CAT scan to make sure everything looks right.

Having major surgeries has taken its toll on her. She keeps saying, "I forgot I came for a heart with everything else that has happened."

The doctors told us yesterday that if everything goes smoothly, we could be home next week!

IT'S TIME,
Lynne

Wednesday, April 23, 2014

Good morning,

We found out we will not be going home this week.
When I woke up a couple of days ago, I noticed Lauren was not breathing right. It looked just like when we were rushed back to the hospital from rehab. I went to get her nurse and told her something was wrong. I knew Lauren was in trouble again. When a person doesn't let out enough carbon dioxide, they are very sleepy, cannot concentrate, pretty much slipping into unconsciousness and gasping for air. We were lucky and caught it before she was in real trouble again. She needed to be on bi-pap to help her body rid itself of the carbon dioxide again. By 2pm, she was back to normal.

We also hit another bump. Her creatinine levels in her kidneys are a little elevated. Her level this morning was 2.77, with normal levels being between 0.5 - 1.1. They have a kidney specialist watching her. When we first met him, my face turned white. He asked me if I was okay and I told him, "I just read your jacket; it says Kidney Transplant." He assured me Lauren is not in need of a transplant.

The plan for Lauren's kidneys: they need to keep making adjustments to her meds to bring her levels down. It seems we get rid of one problem and another one arises. I've been so stressed out about this that this morning when I woke up, my lips were very swollen and red. It looked like I had had a Botox treatment. The nurses asked me what happened and I said "This is what happens when you live in a hospital."

We haven't seen the doctors this morning yet, but yesterday they told us they feel confident that we will be going home next week. I am very nervous about going home. Lauren will be leaving with her trache in sc the doctors told me they ordered a ventilator for the house as well as oxygen. They asked me if I felt comfortable taking care of her with th trache at home. I told them I'll do what I have to do.

Love,
Lynne

197

Ninth Biopsy Results
Wednesday, May 7 2014

NO REJECTION!

This was the best news we've had in a long time. Lauren has only had one rejection and the way the doctors explained it, it was only slight. Not only were we blessed to get a new heart but a heart that Lauren's body needed. I still wonder who gave Lauren this beautiful gift and I hope we can someday thank the family.

Last night Lauren and I were sitting here talking about how long we have been in the hospital. We need a calendar to count but we definitely know it has been more than 365 days total.

When the transplant team came in yesterday, I asked if I could have a Mother's Day wish granted: to be home with my daughter and family. They told me it depends on Lauren's kidneys. Her levels are still a little high so they are changing her medications to bring them down. They told us they would be happy with a 1.7; yesterday she was at 3.53. We'll see what today's numbers say.

The doctor also said something that I thought was so nice; he suggested that every Sunday should be Mother's Day for me. If we can't be home this Sunday, yes, I will be disappointed, but I do know that we will be home soon. Lauren's safety is top priority. I don't want her home until the doctors feel confident she is good to go.

Today is going to be a big day. Lauren is taking her second shower of the year. I'm so excited; it means life is moving forward. Also, today is a big training day for me. We will be going home with her trache so I need to learn how to take care of her along with knowing the proper way to suction her airway. For the past few weeks, the nurses have been training me in everything; taking blood pressure with a manual cuff for instance (I think I finally got it perfected.).

I'll take her pressure and write my numbers down, then the nurse will take it. Nursing School 101 for me.
Lynne

Friday May 9 2014

We received the news we have been waiting for yesterday. Lauren's kidney levels have dropped. Last night her creatinine was 1.44. Thanks to everyone for all the prayers, we really needed them. The doctor told us he would be happy to send Lauren home with a 1.7, so guess what we were told??

THEY ARE GOING TO START MAKING OUR PLANS TO GO HOME!

They still need to get some of her medications adjusted but our lives here at the Brigham's Hotel is going to be over soon. I really think it's going to happen. They plan on taking her Hickman line out on

Monday. A Hickman line is a central line that goes right in to her artery so they can draw blood and administer IV drugs without continually poking her. They would not take this out if we were staying. If I were to take a guess, I would say we will be coming home maybe next Wednesday.

Lauren will be coming home with her trache and feeding tube. I still need to learn how to operate the ventilator; when she sleeps at night she has to be connected to keep moisture inside her trache. During the day she is capped and her stats have been staying at 98% oxygen level. The plan is to have her capped longer each day until she is capped all the time, then the trache can come out. The feeding tube will come out when she is eating enough calories on her own. Her appetite is getting better. At night, she's connected to her feeding machine. I have been taking her to the cafe in the hospital so she can eat what she wants. No hospital food. It's costing me a fortune but all that matters is that she is eating.

My thoughts on going home: scared but excited; it's about time. I know we are going to have a great support team with our visiting nurses and I do feel confident with all my training in the medical field.

Love,
Lynne & Lauren

Chapter 26

GOING HOME

Monday May 12, 2014

THE CAR IS READY

WE ARE GOING HOME TODAY!

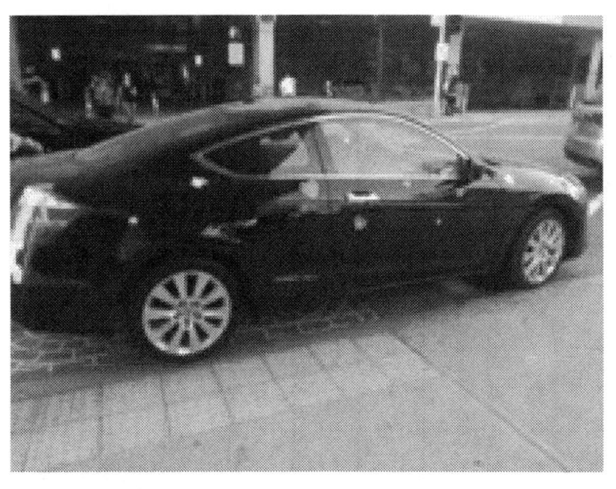

I can't express how I'm feeling. It's been a long, long road but Lauren will now have a new life with a beautiful new heart. I can't thank everyone enough for all the support and prayers during our journey, I wish I could reach out and hug everyone. I decorated my card with all hearts that day for our ride home. I was a proud mother to be bringing my daughter home finally with her new heart.

Time to start the day and get things going.

CHICOPEE MA. HERE WE COMI

THE DAY WE LEFT THE HOSPITAL FOR GOOD!

Standing Outside the Front Doors

I told Lauren we were going to walk out these doors together and we did!

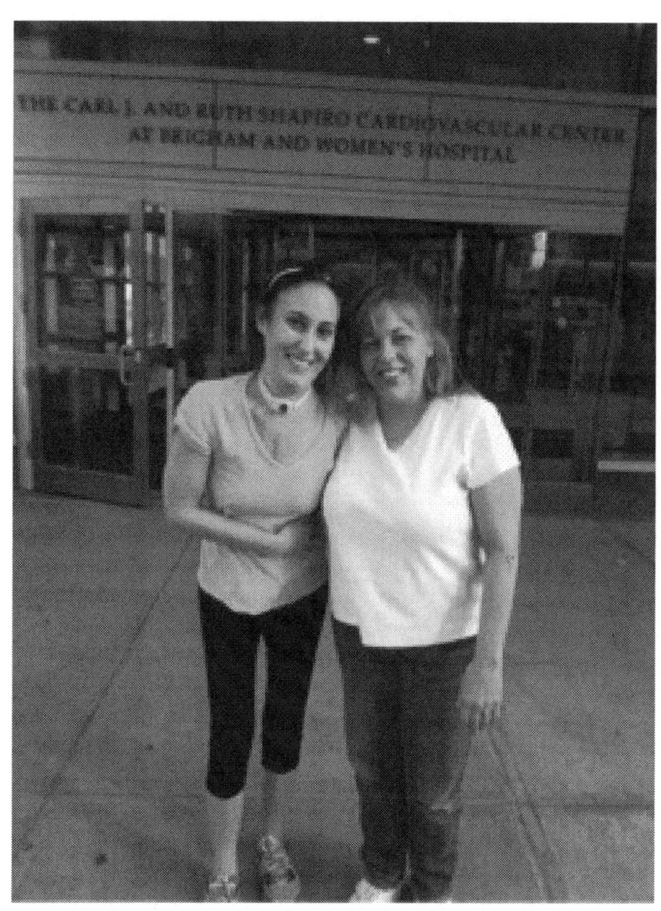

Chapter 27

Time To Get Back to our Lives

June 13, 2014

Home. I still can't believe that we're home. No more hospital living. Time to start a new chapter in our lives.

We've been home for about a month and all I can say is that I'm still a ball of nerves, so afraid that something is going to happen and we'll have to go back to living in a hospital.

Stay positive Lynne, everything is great.

When we arrived home, it was very busy. So much to prepare for. We had a ventilator with tubing brought to the house for her trache. She still has her teach because if she was to get into trouble with her breathing again the hole will already be in place. This is her third trache, she has too much scar tissue from the past tracheotomies so the doctors decided to keep it in to be on the safe side at home. For me that means at night I have to take her cap out and connect her to the ventilator which is on her night stand to keep moisture in the hole. This allows her to breathe easier. Sometimes it will clog up and I have to suction it out and clean it every day. This plays into the nursing training I needed to take.

Lauren is taking 32 pills a day. Managing her meds is a full time job in itself. She has a schedule that the hospital created as to what to take and when. The only problem is, sometimes they make her sick and she will end up throwing them up. If she tries to take them on an empty stomach she won't keep them down. Most of the time in the mornings she isn't hungry so I need to force her to eat a little yogurt. I'm not even going to go into the cost of all her prescriptions, but holy hell. She needs these to live. She'll be on these for the rest of her life. They consist of anti-rejects, vitamins, potassium, magnesium, pain and anxiety meds, Pepsid and Torsemide. We have a pill organizer, otherwise forget about trying to keep track. Every day I take out the day, place it on the table and we know these are the pills she needs to take, broken up for four times a day.

We are what I consider lucky; we have a visiting nurse that comes to the house four times a week to start. The number of visits will decrease when we become comfortable with everything. It brings great peace of mind to have help. Every day I must check Lauren's blood pressure (I have my own cuff and was trained to do this) and I also need to check her blood sugar. I'm very impressed with myself when the nurse comes and I take Lauren's blood pressure, then the nurse will take it to see if we have the same numbers. Spot on. Those are times I'm very proud of myself. Our nurse has become part of our family; we love her so much (I'm talking about you, Dee). Aside from Dee's visits, Lauren has both occupational and physical therapists that come multiple times a week. Her muscles are still very weak and due to her immune system being so severely compromised, she can't go to an outpatient facility yet. But every day she gets a little stronger and in no time she'll be back at the gym pumping iron like she used to! Just baby steps at this time.

As far as it goes, it is nice to be able to do things that we take for granted. Examples: taking a shower, doing laundry to wear clean clothes, opening the fridge to grab something to eat, sitting alone, going outside, driving a car. Just think of everything we do in our lives that is taken away when living in a hospital for a lengthy period of time. For me, I'd have to say the best part is being at home with my family.

Never take things for granted, they could be taken away in an instant.

We don't know who Lauren's heart donor is yet. We really would like to know the family of the angel that saved my daughter's life. The proper etiquette to inquire about your donor is as follows. First you must wait one full year before writing your letter. When it's time to write your letter, you can't put any personal contact about yourself in it. The letter should be about why you want to meet the family. It's then submitted to UNSO and they will read the letter for approval.

Once it's approved, UNSO will forward your letter the family and it'll be up to them if they want to be known; some families do, while othe don't. We really hope we'll find out, but we will have to respect their decision if they don't want to be known.

This has been a journey with a happy ending. My daughter received her gift of life and we will forever be grateful to the donor.

Currently there are 123,000 people on the heart transplant list. Every 10 minutes a person is added to the waiting list while every day 22 people will die while waiting. One organ donor can save the lives of 8 people while enhancing more than 50 lives.

Writing this book, our story has brought back so many memories. It was like I was reliving our journey all over again. It has made me realize not to take life for granted, which is very easy to do; we just get caught up in our everyday lives.

Love and Good Bless

Lynne, Lauren & Dean

May 10, 2017

Message From Lauren

Hi everyone,

It's been a little over 4 years since my journey to my new heart began and I can't believe how good I feel! When I went for my 3-year annual appointment in December, I received the best cardiac report I've have yet. My heart isn't as stiff as it was, all my numbers were normal, and my body hasn't been rejecting the heart. It feels amazing going to the doctors now and not having to worry if/when I'll be leaving.

Despite all the good news now, I have had a few more surgeries since my last entry three years ago. I've had my trache hole revised, so now it's flat and can easily be hidden with makeup. The scar on the back of my head has been fixed too. My plastic surgeon ended u cutting the scar out and pulling the skin together, a 'backwards facelift' as we call it. At least when I'm 60, I'll look 40 :)

In January of 2016, I had a fistula surgery performed in my groin. A fistula is when your vein and artery get connected (mine was due to all the biopsies) and the oxygenated and deoxygenated blood mix. This was causing the pressure in my heart to sky rocket. The doctor thought I only had one but I never make things easy: I had three. One friend of mine jokes and says surgeries are a hobby of mine!

Every day I get a little stronger. I'm still in physical therapy, for I'm what they call a 'maintenance patient.' With my muscular dystrophy, I go for a couple months then I stop for a few until I start back up.

This allows me to go a full year without running out of sessions with the insurance company.

I'm back to the gym too! I go a few times a week, which feels great. Three years ago when I was crying, 'I can't do it' while trying to walk, I never thought I'd be doing three miles on a treadmill. I see how my physical endurance is improving, allowing myself to keep up with my friends.

As for my mental state, I still see a therapist to help me cope. Some days are worse than others and I suffer from PTSD but I'm realizing how lucky I am and how far I've come. I look back at pictures or read old entries and I can't believe that was me. Man, did I look like hell!

I still learn something new all the time about that chapter of my life. For example, the other day I asked Mom if I'd cried when they were wheeling me into surgery. She said, 'Nope! You were on your knees, giving everyone hugs and kisses with a smile on your face, just wanting to get it done and over with. Granted, you had some good meds in you already!' Hearing things like that, of how strong I was makes me happy. I'm just proud of myself that I got through it and I truly am as strong as people say.

Currently, I'm an ambassador for Donate Life and a Leading Lady for the American Heart Association. Spreading the importance of organ donation and heart disease has become a new passion of mine. Unfortunately it took me being on my death bed to realize how precious life is and how quickly it can be taken away.

I only had to wait 9 months to get my heart, while others wait longer and some may never even get the call. I'm proud and grateful at the same time that my Mom kept a blog and then took the time to turn it into a book. The organ donation process isn't like how you see in the movies. There isn't a supply of organs kept in a special room just waiting for someone who needs it.

YOU need to sign up and become an organ donor. It could potentially save someone's life.

With that chapter of my life done, I can't wait to see what life has in store for me. I'd like to say thank you, Mom for always being there for me, as well as writing a book based on our journey. I know what I went through as the patient but I can't imagine what you went through as a mother. YOU are the strongest person I know and I love you.

I hope one day we can meet the family of the angel who gave me a second chance at life...

Love always,

Lauren M. Meizo

Helpful Suggestions if you find yourself living in a Hospital

During my time living in the hospital for close to a year and a half, I would like to pass on a few helpful suggestions for anyone that might be in the same situation. Keep in mind all hospitals are different, with their own rules and requirements.

- You are going to feel overwhelmed (that's an understatement) so organization will help you stay focused. Get yourself a binder with at least twenty folders with tabs. Label each folder, for example: doctors, procedures, health care proxy, consent forms, insurance papers, work papers, etc. It will be very helpful to have everything you need in one spot. Easy referral.

- Social Worker - A social worker will give the patient, and also their family, emotional support and help everyone cope with hospitalization. They also help with insurance or financial issues. I found there was nothing I couldn't ask our social worker; they really want to help.

- Parking Passes - Most hospitals will give out vouchers for long-term parking for the families.

- Meal Vouchers - Eating can be very expensive in a hospital; me vouchers do exist.

-

- Laundry Services - Yes, some hospitals have coin-operated washers and dryers for you to use.

- Sleeping arrangements - Depending on the hospital, I was able to stay with my daughter at all times. I was able to bring in my own bedding to make it as comfortable as possible for the couch. I even brought in a small table fan to feel air circulating.

- Salon - Some hospitals do have a salon in the building, with hairdressers that will come to your room. A new hairdo or haircut can go a long way, not only physically but also emotionally.

- If you are going to be long term, you can ask for a small refrigerator for your room.

- This one is important: you can talk with the floor manager if you feel a nurse is not giving the care the patient requires. Also, some people just don't mesh; it happens. You do have the right to request that a nurse not be in charge of your care.

- Get to know your surrounding areas outside the hospital. Example: drug stores, if you need to fill prescriptions yourself, restaurants just to get out, and also to know where you can

- To help pass time, I started to crochet. I made a blanket for my daughter and granddaughter. It helped to keep my mind and hands busy.

- Keep a journal. I would like to write in the morning with my cup of coffee. It gave me a routine; you need something to look forward to.

Many different states have different regulations and agencies. If you are taking care of a sick person, you may be considered a caregiver. There are agencies that will pay you to do this job, even for a family member

* Cardiovascular Center, Brigham and Womens Faulkner Hospital

Made in the USA
Middletown, DE
20 October 2018